Immune Responses to Metastases

Volume I

Editors

Ronald B. Herberman, M.D.
Director
Pittsburgh Cancer Institute
and
Professor of Medicine and Pathology
University of Pittsburgh
Pittsburgh, Pennsylvania

Robert H. Wiltrout, Ph.D.
Head
Experimental Therapeutics Section
Laboratory of Experimental
Immunology
Biological Response Modifiers Program
Division of Cancer Treatment
National Cancer Institute
Frederick, Maryland

Elieser Gorelik, M.D.
Investigator
Pittsburgh Cancer Institute
and
Associate Professor of Pathology
University of Pittsburgh
Pittsburgh, Pennsylvania

CRC Press, Inc.
Boca Raton, Florida

Library of Congress Cataloging-in-Publication Data

Immune responses to metastases.

Includes bibliographies and index.
1. Metastasis—Immunological aspects.
2. Immunotherapy.   I. Herberman, Ronald B., 1940-
II. Wiltrout, Robert H.   III. Gorelik, Elieser.
[DNLM: 1. Neoplasm Metastasis—immunology.   2. Neoplasm
Metastasis—therapy.   QZ 202 I325]
RC268.3.I44   1987   616.99′4071   86-7878
ISBN 0-8493-5847-7 (v. 1)
ISBN 0-8493-5848-5 (v. 2)
ISBN 0-8493-5849-3 (set)

Direct all inquiries to CRC Press, Inc., 2000 Corporate Blvd., N.W., Boca Raton, Florida, 33431.

© 1987 by CRC Press, Inc.

International Standard Book Number 0-8493-5847-7 (v. 1)
International Standard Book Number 0-8493-5848-5 (v. 2)
International Standard Book Number 0-8493-5849-3 (set)

Library of Congress Card Number 86-7878
Printed in the United States

PREFACE

The greatest limitation to the successful treatment of cancer is the ability of tumors to form distant metastases. These metastases are often located in vital organs and are either inaccessible or refractory to conventional forms of cancer treatment. In addition, primary tumors and their metastases are often composed of subpopulations or foci of tumor cells that differ in their sensitivity to the various forms of cancer treatment. This heterogeneity within a tumor cell population contributes appreciably to the inability of chemotherapeutic drugs or radiotherapy to completely eradicate established tumors and thereby cure rather than just delay the progression of the disease. A further limitation of conventional cancer treatment is the necessity to balance the toxicity of chemotherapy or irradiation for the patient with the dose-dependent beneficial antitumor effects of these modalities. Therefore, the ideal form of cancer therapy would be selective for the tumor and thereby nontoxic to the host, able to circumvent heterogeneity within a given tumor, and be able to reach tumor metastases in all anatomical sites. Based on these criteria, high expectations have arisen that the immune system can be explited as a weapon against cancer, and more specifically against metastases. The rationale for these high expectations is based on the exquisite specificity associated with T-lymphocytes and antibodies, the broad yet tumor selective cytotoxic activity of NK cells, LAK cells and macrophages, and the presence of these effector mechanisms in most organs and anatomical compartments. In order for immunologic approaches to the treatment of cancer to live up to their expected potential, it seems essential to systematically investigate the parameters required for optimal stimulation of effector activities and for selective accumulation of effector cells and/or molecules at the sites of metastases. This should provide the needed foundation for the rational design of therapeutic trials in experimental tumor systems and in patients with cancer.

In this volume, we have summarized the current status of the field and have attempted to identify major issues for future investigaitons. In particular, we have addressed three aspects of the relationship between the host immune system and tumor metastases. First, because the process of metastasis is complex, several chapters (Chapters 1 to 3) have been included to address various aspects of the metastatic phenotype which related to host-tumor interactions. These contributions summarize the evidence that considerable heterogeneity exists within metastatic tumor cell populations and illustrate the ways in which this heterogeneity influences, and is influenced by, the immune system. Secondly, the interaction between the immune system and metastases is bidirectional. Therefore, we have included contributions which are at least partially devoted to summarizing the impact of metastasis formation and tumor progression on various components of the immune system and the ways in which different parameters of immunity change in response to tumor growth (Chapters 1 to 7). Thirdly, and most central to the ultimate objective of this field or research, considerable attention is focused on approaches to modulating and utilizing host immunity for the express purpose of preventing or eradicating metastases (Chapter 8 to 14).

Overall, the chapters in this volume demonstrate that many advances have been made in understanding the metastatic process and host-tumor interactions. Further, significant advances have also been made with regard to modulation of immunity and our understanding of how to optimize this modulation. These insights already have translated into considerable progress in the development of successful strategies for the immunotherapy of experimental metastases. However, the successful application of these approaches to the treatment of human cancer remains to be developed. In the clinical trials with immunotherapy of metastases which are now being planned or are underway, it would seem important if not essential to follow the principles elucidated in these experimental systems, in order to optimize the potential of these approaches for the cure of human cancer.

THE EDITORS

Ronald B. Herberman, M.D., is Director of the Pittsburgh Cancer Institute and Professor of Medicine and Pathology at the University of Pittsburgh, Pennsylvania.

Dr. Herberman received his undergraduate and doctoral education at New York University, receiving a B.A. degree in 1960 and a M.D. degree in 1964. He then served as an intern and resident in internal medicine at the Massachusetts General Hospital from 1964 to 1966. He then went to the National Cancer Institute as a Clinical Associate in 1966 and then progressed to a series of positions of increasing responsibility, including Head of the Cellular and Tumor Immunology section of the Laboratory of Cell Biology, Chief of the Laboratory of Immunodiagnosis, and then Chief of the Biological Therapeutics Branch in the Biological Response Modifiers Program. In addition, during his last year at the National Cancer Institute he was Acting Associate Director for the Biological Response Modifiers Program. In 1985, he moved to Pittsburgh to begin the organization of a new cancer center, associated both with the University of Pittsburgh, Carnegie-Mellon University, and the University Health Center of Pittsburgh.

Dr. Herberman is a member of the American Association of Immunologists, American Association for Cancer Research, American Federation for Clinical Research, American Society for Clinical Investigation, Transplantation Society, and Reticuloendothelial Society. He is a Fellow of the American College of Physicians and of the American Academy of Microbiology. He was elected President of the Reticuloendothelial Society in 1984. He was awarded a commendation medal from the United States Public Health Service.

Dr. Herberman is the author of more than 600 papers and has been the Editor of six books. His current major research interests relate to cellular and tumor immunology and the use of immunological approaches for the diagnosis and therapy of cancer.

Robert H. Wiltrout, Ph.D., is Head of the Experimental Therapeutics Section at the Biological Response Modifiers Program of the National Cancer Institute's Frederick Cancer Research Facility, Frederick, Maryland. Dr. Wiltrout received his B.A. from Kutztown University, Kutztown, Pennsylvania, his M.S. from the Pennsylvania State University, University Park, Pennsylvania, and his Ph.D. from the Wayne State University School of Medicine, Detroit, Michigan.

Dr. Wiltrout is a member of several professional organizations, including the Reticuloendothelial Society, The American Association of Immunologists, and the Honorary Society Sigma Xi. He has published more than 90 articles, contributions to books, and abstracts. His current research interests include the biology of metastasis and the application of biological response modifiers to the treatment of cancer.

Elieser Gorelik, M.D., Ph.D. was born in the USSR. He graduated from the State Medical School, Minsk, USSR in 1961 and received his Ph.D. degree in 1968 from the Institute of Genetics and Cytology, Byelorussian Academy of Science. In 1975, he emigrated to Israel and worked at the Weizmann Institute of Science. In 1979, he was invited to come to the National Cancer Institute, National Institutes of Health, where he has worked until recently. He has just now initiated research at the Pittsburgh Cancer Institute. Dr. Gorelik is the author of about 100 articles, of which 70 were published after his emigration.

Dr. Gorelik is a member of several professional organizations, including the American Association for Cancer Research. His research interests relate to tumor immunology and investigation of the role of the immune system in the control of metastatic spread and growth.

CONTRIBUTORS

Paola Allavena, M.D.
Research Associate
Mario Negri Institute for
  Pharmacological Research
Milan, Italy

Peter Altevogt, Ph.D.
Associate Member
Institute Immunologie and Genetik
Deutsches Krebsforschungszentr
Heidelberg, West Germany

Malcolm George Baines, Ph.D.
Associate Professor
Department of Microbiology and
  Immunology
McGill University
Montreal, Quebec, Canada

Claudia Balotta, M.D.
Research Assistant
Mario Negri Institute for
  Pharmacological Research
Milan, Italy

Barbara Bottazzi, Ph.D.
Research Associate
Mario Negri Institute for
  Pharmacological Research
Milan, Italy

Jorge A. Carrasquillo, M.D.
Attending Physician
Department of Nuclear Medicine
National Institutes of Health
Bethesda, Maryland

Isaiah J. Fidler, D.V.M., Ph.D.
R. E. "Bob" Smith Chair in Cell
  Biology
Professor and Chairman
Department of Cell Biology
M.D. Anderson Hospital and Tumor
  Institute
Houston, Texas

William E. Fogler, Ph.D.
Research Scientist
Department of Membrane Biochemistry
Walter Reed Army Institute of
  Research
Washington, D.C.

Elieser Gorelik, M.D., Ph.D.
Investigator
Pittsburgh Cancer Institute
Associate Professor of Pathology
University of Pittsburgh
Pittsburgh, Pennsylvania

Michael G. Hanna, Jr., Ph.D.
Vice President and Director
Research and Development
Bionetics Research, Inc.
Rockville, Maryland

Nabil Hanna, Ph.D.
Director
Department of Immunology
Smith Kline and French Laboratories
Swedeland, Pennsylvania

Ruediger Heicappell, M.D.
Guest Scientist
Institute Immunologie and Genetik
Deutsches Krebsforschungszentrum
Heidelberg, West Germany

Ingegerd Hellström, M.D.
Vice President and Laboratory Director
Oncogene
University of Washington
Seattle, Washington

Karl Erik Hellström, M.D.
Vice President and Laboratory Director
Oncogene
University of Washington
Seattle, Washington

Gloria H. Heppner, Ph.D.
Scientific Director
Research Division
Michigan Cancer Foundation
Detroit, Michigan

Ronald B. Herberman, M.D.
Director
Pittsburgh Cancer Institute
and
Professor of Medicine and Pathology
University of Pittsburgh
Pittsburgh, Pennsylvania

Herbert C. Hoover, Jr., M.D.
Chief, Surgical Oncology
Division of Surgical Oncology
State University of New York, Stony
  Brook
Stony Brook, New York

Steven M. Larson, M.D.
Chief
Nuclear Medicine Department
National Institutes of Health
Bethesda, Maryland

Alberto Mantovani, M.D.
Chief
Laboratory of Human Immunology
Mario Negri Institute for
  Pharmacological Research
Milan, Italy

Fred R. Miller, Ph.D.
Associate Member
Department of Immunology
Research Division
Michigan Cancer Foundation
Detroit, Michigan

James J. Mulé, Ph.D.
Senior Staff Fellow
Surgery Branch
National Cancer Institute
National Institutes of Health
Bethesda, Maryland

David S. Nelson, D.Sc., F.R.A.C.P.
Director
Kolling Institute of Medical Research
The Royal North Shore Hospital of
  Sydney
St. Leonards, New South Wales,
  Australia

Garth L. Nicolson, Ph.D.
Florence M. Thomas Professor
  Cancer Research
Chairman
Department of Tumor Biology
University of Texas
M.D. Anderson Hosptial and Tumor
  Institute
Houston, Texas

Susan M. North, Ph.D.
Research Associate
Department of Tumor Biology
University of Texas
M.D. Anderson Hospital and Tumor
  Institute
Houston, Texas

Hugh F. Pross, M.D., Ph.D., F.R.C.P
Professor and Head
Department of Radiation Oncology,
  Microbiology, and Immunology
Queen's University
Kingston, Ontario, Canada

Steven A. Rosenberg, M.D., Ph.D.
Chief of Surgery
Surgery Branch
National Cancer Institute
National Institute of Health
Bethesda, Maryland

Volker Schirrmacher, Ph.D.
Head
Professor
Department of Cellular Immunology
Institute Immunologie and Genetik
Deutches Krebsforschungszentrum
Heidelberg, West Germany

James E. Talmadge
Head
Preclinical Screening Laboratory
Program Resources, Inc.
NCI-Frederick Cancer Research Facility
Frederick, Maryland

P. von Hoegen, Ph.D.
Student
Institute Immunologie and Genetik
Deutsches Krebsforschungzentru
Heidelberg, West Germany

Robert H. Wiltrout, Ph.D.
Head
Experimental Therapeutics Section
Laboratory of Experimental
  Immunology
Biological Response Modifiers Program
Division of Cancer Treatment
NCI-Frederick Cancer Research Facility
Frederick, Maryland

TABLE OF CONTENTS

VOLUME I

VOLUME II

Chapter 1

HOST RESPONSES AND TUMOR METASTASIS

Susan M. North and Garth L. Nicolson

TABLE OF CONTENTS

I. INTRODUCTION

The spread of malignant tumor cells from primary sites to near and distant secondary sites is one of the most important events in the pathogenesis of cancer. It is this process that accounts for the majority of deaths from cancer. Although most primary tumors can be treated successfully by surgery alone or in combination with other therapeutic procedures, the therapy of metastases has proved to be a more difficult and complex problem. This is so because at the time of diagnosis a large proportion of patients already have multiple metastases, many of which are undetectable by currently available imaging and laboratory procedures. Even when such micrometastases can be detected, methods like surgical resection may be impossible to apply.

Metastatic cells are often very diverse in their properties and metastatic potentials. Such diversity encompasses differences in the expression of cell surface glycoproteins, glycolipids, antigens, enzymes, and receptors, and in the release of these components, as well as known differences in cell morphology, karyotype, and histochemical properties. Of major importance is the extensive variation of individual metastatic cells in sensitivity to therapeutic agents, such as drugs, radiation, and hyperthermia, and to host-response mechanisms (reviewed in References 1 to 6).

Cellular heterogeneity is not strictly a property of malignant neoplasms; it occurs also in normal cells but usually not to the same extent. Although normal tissues may maintain relatively stable cellular phenotypes, they are also heterogeneous in the expression of particular properties.[7-9]

The origin of metastatic cells and highly malignant cell subpopulations is unknown, although they are apt to arise spontaneously during the progressive growth of malignant neoplasms subjected to various host-selection pressures. In time this process tends to generate tumors that contain phenotypically diverse cell subpopulations. Foulds[10-12] described the process as neoplastic evolution during which each tumor gradually gains autonomy from its host while at the same time acquiring certain cellular characteristics. Virtually any tumor characteristic is subject to variation and host-selection, which leads to the evolution of cellular diversity during progressive tumor growth. The result of these changes is the gradual escape of cells from growth controls and regulatory processes of the host that attempt to restrain the emergence of the more malignant tumor cell phenotypes.

The evolution and progression of tumors, accompanied by the emergence of varied tumor cell subpopulations with altered malignant and other properties has been proposed to be caused by genetic alterations.[13] Tumor cells that have diversified rapidly, for example, should display enhanced genetic instability and eventually acquire the properties most favorable for survival, growth, and malignancy under constant host-selection pressures. This hypothesis is supported by cytogenetic and genetic data that indicate that gross chromosomal alterations, mitotic errors, and spontaneous mutations in highly malignant cells occur at higher rates than in normal cells or those with low malignant potential.[14-17]

The theories of Foulds[10-12] and Nowell,[13,14] which advanced the concept that tumor cell progression is the result of increased genetic alterations generated by random somatic mutation, cannot explain the rapid rate of tumor diversification seen in many malignant neoplasms. This is because the highest known rates of spontaneous gene mutation in highly metastatic cells, such as 5 to 7×10^{-5}/cell/generation found by Cifone and Fidler,[17] are a magnitude lower than the rates of phenotypic variation found in many malignant systems. Extremely rapid rates of cell-variant generation, as high as 10^{-2}/cell/generation, have been observed in a variety of tumors.[18-22] This led to the proposal that phenotypic diversification is generated by alterations in gene structure or chromosomal arrangements or integration of viral sequences.[14,23,24]

Although permanent genetic changes undoubtedly occur during tumor progression, there is also evidence for the belief that tumor cell heterogeneity is also generated by reversible changes in gene expression. In an attempt to understand more fully the nature of tumor heterogeneity, clones of cells have been isolated from a number of tumor models.[25-28] These studies demonstrated the phenotypic instability of tumor cell clones and the rapid regeneration of antigenic heterogeneity.[28,29]

Host-tumor interactions seem to occur largely at the level of the cell surface.[3-5,15,23,24] This has stimulated investigators to examine the cell surface properties of metastatic tumors, as well as cell sublines and clones with differing metastatic properties.[30-32] Although differences in certain cell surface properties have correlated with differences in the metastatic behavior of particular cell clones, some of these findings have been equivocal, probably because of the high probability that heterogeneity is rapidly generated by cellular instability during the clonal expansion required for such studies.

In addition to genetic changes that may occur in tumor cells, such epigenetic mechanisms as nonmutational DNA modifications may offer additional mechanisms for generating phenotypic instability. For example, modifications in DNA methylation by 5-aza-cytidine can result in the rapid modulation of tumor cell phenotypes.[33]

Finally, the role of tumor microenvironment in influencing cellular phenotypic instabilities is believed to be important.[15,23,34] The microenvironment of individual cells within a tumor is unique because of variabilities in the concentrations of nutrients, such as oxygen, growth hormones, enzymes, ions, inducers, and other regulatory molecules (Figure 1). These and other differences in various conditions and agents could lead to phenotypic diversification of tumor cell subpopulations. Cells and tissues are normally regulated by a variety of microenvironmental signals that control normal cellular differentiation. As tumors progress, their abilities to be regulated by stromal components and soluble factors may change.[35-37] In addition, some tumors show extensive infiltration by such normal host cells as lymphocytes, granulocytes, and macrophages. Since the interactions of host cells with tumor cells will be discussed in detail in subsequent chapters of this monograph it suffices here to mention that normal host cells may have profound effects on tumor growth and phenotypic properties.

II. HOST RESPONSES AND METASTASIS

That both specific and nonspecific host responses against growing tumors influence the outcome of neoplastic disease is not doubted; but whether effective host antitumor mechanisms can operate in vivo and which ones are most important are still debated. This is probably because intensive studies are being done with numerous animal tumor models of differing etiologies, and some of the findings are being inappropriately extended to human cancers. It is apparent that, in many metastatic animal tumor models, manipulation of immune systems may result in either increased or decreased metastases.[38-42] These disparate results have led to severe criticisms of the use of highly immunogenic, chemically or virally induced tumors as experimental systems for evaluating the relative importance of host immunity in tumor growth and metastasis.[43,44]

The history of the use of highly immunogenic, chemically or virally induced tumors has been described by many workers.[45-48] With the use of such tumors, investigators hoped to establish the existence and specificity of tumor-associated transplantation antigens (TATA). It has been argued, however, that human cancers do not possess TATA, and such tumors are thought to be only weakly immunogenic in the autochthonous host.[43] The use of "spontaneous" tumors, those that arise in the animal population without deliberate carcinogenic stimuli, has been advocated as an experimental model that is more relevant to the pathogenesis of the disease in humans. In general, these spontaneous animal tumors are not highly immunogenic.[43] Some currently under

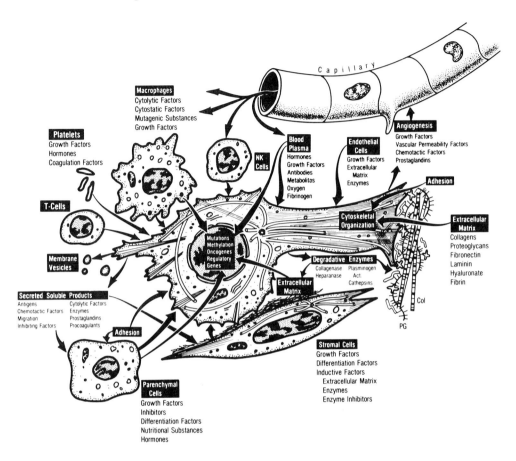

FIGURE 1. Microenvironmental influences on malignant tumor cells. Soluble components, cells, extracellular matrix, and other factors affect individual tumor cells differentially. (Reproduced with permission from Nicolson, G. L., *Cancer Metastasis Rev.,* 3, 25, 1984.)

examination elicit no detectable immune response, but, unfortunately, the behavior of human cancers is not so predictable, and the immunogenicity of human tumors cannot be measured by the same criteria as those established for animal models. Although other mechanisms may exist, the late development of some human cancers infers that host resistance may occur as in, for example, the long-term growth dormancy of certain metastases.[49-51]

To rationalize the disparate effects of host immunity on metastasis Prehn[52] proposed that more than one competing host immune mechanism is likely to be involved in antitumor responses and that some responses could stimulate rather than inhibit tumor growth. Although the hypothesis of immunostimulation is tantalizing, it is difficult to prove or disprove.[53] Prehn suggested that a weak, stimulatory antitumor response occurs at the early stages of tumor development, or in weakly antigenic tumors, but at the later stages of tumor development, or in cases where the tumors are highly antigenic, a strong inhibitory response develops. Although speculative, some support for this hypothesis has been gathered.[54,55]

In early attempts to discover the nature of TATA and their relationship to metastasis, the chemically or virally induced tumors that were used showed them to be highly immunogenic. However, a number of investigations have found differences in the immunogenicity of spontaneously arising tumors growing at a primary site and the immunogenicity of their metastases.[56-60] Kim[60] demonstrated, for example, that metastatic mammary carcinomas were less immunogenic or lost immunogenicity compared to their nonmetastatic counterparts. There are numerous reports in which inhibition of metastasis by immunologic means was successfully achieved with experimental tumor models in which the antigenic determinants recognized were TATA,[61-63] viral antigens,[64] or oncofetal antigens.[65,66] These data suggested that metastatic tumor cells can differ from primary tumor cells in the type, amount, or display of cell surface antigens.

Cell surface antigenic variation has been shown to be related to the metastatic capability of specific tumors. For example, Reading et al.[64] reported a direct correlation between increased metastatic potential and loss of cell surface glycoprotein gp70 from cell sublines and clones of the murine RAW117 lymphosarcoma. In this system decreases in viral gp70 expression correlated with increased liver colonization. One can postulate that, at least in this animal tumor model, successful colonization required escape from host immune surveillance through antigen deletion. Subsequent studies indicated that the effector cells necessary for this selection were probably tumoricidal macrophages.[67] Fogel et al.[58] also found a correlation between antigen loss and metastatic potential.

The demonstration of unique antigens on the surfaces of tumor cells in experimental animals encouraged similar work with human tumors, in which tumor-associated antigens were expected to be found and isolated. Evidence obtained in the early 1970s suggested that tumor-associated antigens (TAA) were present in the serum of patients with malignant disease,[68] and more recent data, particularly from the use of monoclonal antibodies documented the heterogeneity of human neoplasms with respect to antigenic variation of primary tumors and their metastases.[69] There appears to be no real correlation, however, between metastatic potential and loss or acquisition of particular cell surface antigens.

The generation in vivo of antigen loss variants implies that TAA are immunogenic and can elicit an immune response capable of eliminating most malignant cells, resulting in the survival of a highly selected cell population. Acquisition of either "new" antigens or increased expression of existing antigens could be important for specific events during metastasis such as blood-borne implantation. Indeed, recent data from our laboratory suggest that, in one model for breast cancer, (the 13762NF rat mammary adenocarcinoma), such a selection has occurred. Cloned sublines of this tumor were isolated and characterized from either the primary implant growing subcutaneously in the mammary fat pad or from spontaneous metastases.[28] These cell clones were found to be heterogeneous in a number of properties, but none of these correlated with metastatic potential.[70-72] The only property that showed a positive correlation with metastatic behavior was the increased expression of a high molecular weight mucin-like glycoprotein, gp580.[73] Immune manipulation of recipients of this tumor has demonstrated that the most metastatic tumor cells are not highly immunogenic and appear refractory to manipulation of the immune system in vivo.[74] It is possible that the presence of a high molecular weight mucin-like molecule may have a protective function on 13762NF cells, preventing immune attack on the metastatic cell subpopulation.

It is well known that traumatizing the host with, for example, surgery or anesthesia, may suppress host immunologic defenses against metastases. Using the 13762NF mammary adenocarcinoma model, we demonstrated that removal of the draining inguinal and axillary lymph nodes has a significant effect on the ability of the primary tumor to metastasize. Removal of the lymph nodes 5 days before injection of the tumors resulted in reduced metastases, but removal at 5 days postinjection resulted in extensive metastasis to sites not usually involved, such as the contralateral nodes.[74] These results suggested an immunosuppressive effect by the tumor on host responses (Table 1).

In the discussion to follow it is assumed that the host plays an important role in

Table 1

EFFECT OF LYMPHADENECTOMY ON THE SPONTANEOUS METASTASIS
OF 13762NF (CLONE MTLn3) MAMMARY TUMOR CELLS

Time of treatment (days)	Av. tumor diameter (mm ± SD)	Metastases (No. animals with metastases/total no. animals)						
		Lung	Inguinal nodes	Axillary nodes	Lumbar nodes	Renal nodes	Other	(Location)
−5 sham	13.45 ± 3.40	6/9	9/9	4/9	5/9	0/9	0/9	
−5	13.33 ± 3.48	2/10*	R	R	2/10	2/10	1/10	(Thymus)
							1/10	(Mesentery)
							1/10	(Cervical)
							2/10	(Subaxillary)
−1 sham	21.44 ± 4.17	4/9	5/9	6/9	1/9	0/9	0/9	
−1	22.50 ± 3.85	2/9	R	R(1/9)	0/9	0/9	0/9	
+5 sham	21.72 ± 4.42	4/9	9/9	8/9	6/9	3/9	3/9	(Thymus)
			(1/9)	(2/9)	(2/9)	(1/9)	1/9	(Mesentery)
							2/9	(Cervical)
							2/9	(Illiac)
+5	23.80 ± 6.11	5/9	R(1/9)	R(1/9)	3/9	0/9	0/9	

Note: R = lymph nodes removed; ( ) = lymph node metastases on the contralateral side; and * = all metastases from the same two animals.

determining metastatic properties and can respond effectively against certain metastatic cells.[75,76] One characteristic that may allow malignant cells to accomplish metastasis more effectively, however, is their ability to circumvent host barriers, both immune- and nonimmune-related. Obviously, the malignant cells that can evade host antitumor mechanisms will have a greater chance of survival and growth at secondary sites, and this will be considered along with evidence indicating that host responses can play potentially important roles in the prevention of metastatic disease.

III. CELL-MEDIATED HOST MECHANISMS AGAINST METASTASES

A. Macrophages

The ability of a tumor cell to metastasize is determined by a multitude of tumor cell and host properties.[2-5,23,24] Here we will consider only some of the properties related to host response and some related to tumor microenvironment. Given the complexity of the host, the variety of immune mechanisms that may be brought to bear on individual malignant cells, and the delicate homeostatic balance which exists between various "arms" of the host response mechanisms, it is easy to see that any one explanation for the ability or inability of malignant cells to metastasize is naive. For clarity however, in discussing the potential of host mechanisms in preventing or augmenting metastasis, we will treat them as if they were predominantly separate entities capable of responding effectively against metastatic cells.

Since most of the current information on host mechanisms and metastasis comes from experimental animal tumor systems, not human cancer, our discussion will be somewhat limited, and the reader is referred to the more extensive reviews in this monograph. One aspect of the host defense system that has received particular attention recently is the tumoricidal macrophage.[7*] In some experimental systems, the extent of tumor infiltration by cells of the macrophage/monocyte lineage was found to correlate not only with tumor growth but also with the capacity of such tumors to metastasize.[78-81] Such in vivo studies indicated that a low macrophage content was correspondingly associated with increased metastatic potential; however, other investigators[82,83] failed to find this correlation. Moreover, Mahoney and Heppner[84] demonstrated in their experimental system that macrophage maturity, as assessed by the expression of ectoenzymes, is more important than simple macrophage infiltration. Studies carried out on human tumors seemed to show a distinct mononuclear infiltration, but correlations between metastatic potential and mononuclear infiltration have not been definitively established.[85,86]

Although the presence of infiltrating macrophages in tumor deposits both at primary and secondary sites has been documented, it has been more difficult to prove the actual tumoricidal nature of these cells. Since most tumors progress and do not regress, it has been argued that such tumor-infiltrating macrophages do not play a significant role in preventing either primary tumor growth or metastasis and are in effect "innocent bystanders". One attempt to demonstrate the significance of tumor-infiltrating macrophages in metastatic processes was to deplete the host of macrophages. The consequence of this manipulation was a significant reduction in the number of infiltrating macrophages, concomitant with an increase in pulmonary metastases.[87] In experiments where antibodies have been shown to inhibit tumor growth in vivo, macrophages appear to be involved. In fact, the suppression of tumor growth in vivo by antibody was shown to correlate with the availability of activated macrophages.[88,89]

Most of the data available on the ability of macrophages to kill tumor cells have been derived from in vitro cytotoxicity tests. Evans and Alexander[90] were among the first to demonstrate a direct effect of macrophages on tumor cells in vitro. Since these initial studies, other investigators found that activated macrophages can kill metastatic cells, inhibit their growth in vitro, or both. Stimulation of tumoricidal macrophages and the abilities of such host cells to kill metastatic tumor cells have been proposed to be independent of other tumor cell properties and other host-mediated antitumor mechanisms.

There is good evidence that tumor cells are heterogeneous in their sensitivities to macrophage-mediated cytolysis and/or cytostasis.[91-96] Using the B16 melanoma system, Miner et al.[93] examined the macrophage sensitivities of highly metastatic B16 sublines selected for brain or lung colonization. They found that the B16-B14b line, which preferentially colonizes brain meninges and is also more metastatic to other sites than the parental B16, was much less susceptible to the cytotoxic or cytostatic effects of macrophages or macrophage cytokines released by monocytic tumor cell lines in culture. Similar experiments using RAW117 lymphosarcoma sublines and clones demonstrated that highly metastatic RAW117 cells were more resistant to the cytotoxic and cytostatic effects of activated peritoneal macrophages.[94] Other investigators using either metastatic murine sarcoma[97] or murine mammary adenocarcinoma[98] cell variants came to similar conclusions.

Recently these observations have been extended with another experimental tumor model, the 13762NF mammary tumor, which metastasizes spontaneously to regional lymph nodes and lung. We examined the susceptibility of metastatic 13762NF tumor cell populations to macrophage-mediated cytolysis.[96] A major difference in these studies from others was that we used tumor cell populations isolated from in vivo growing tumors as well as cultured cell lines. We also used intratumoral macrophages in addition to activated peritoneal exudate cells (PECs). A comparison of the lytic ability of PECs and intratumoral macrophages showed that, although the latter cells were tumoricidal after in vitro activation with lipopolysaccharide, the PECs were always more cytolytic on a per-cell basis. Heterogeneity in macrophage killing among the various sublines of the 13762NF adenocarcinoma was complex and depended on tumor cell source. When we used established cultured cell lines as the tumor targets for macrophage-mediated cytolysis, there was little difference in susceptibility. Significant differences in cytolytic activities against various 13762NF cells were seen, however, when

Table 2

IN VITRO CYTOLYSIS OF 13762NF TUMOR EXPLANTS BY ACTIVATED PERITONEAL AND INTRATUMORAL MACROPHAGES

Tumor	Passage[a]	Effector population[b]	Effector: target ratio	cpm	% of cytolysis[c]	Significance[d]
MTLn3	T18, P1	PEC	10:1	8,484 ± 96[e]	21.0[f]	0.001
		PEC	5:1	9,025 ± 403	16.0	
		IT	10:1	9,614 ± 468	11.0[f]	
		IT	5:1	9,769 ± 560	9.0	
		None	0	10,798 ± 560		
MTLn2	T42, P1	PEC	10:1	5,235 ± 544	43.5[f]	0.020
		PEC	5:1	7,219 ± 917	23.0	
		IT	10:1	5,665 ± 181	39.0[f]	
		IT	5:1	7,453 ± 607	19.5	
		None	0	9,257 ± 1,064		
MTF7	T18, P1	PEC	10:1	2,933 ± 148	63.5[f]	0.001
		PEC	5:1	5,643 ± 757	30.0	
		IT	10:1	6,764 ± 177	16.0	
		IT	5:1	7,116 ± 174	11.5	
		None	0	8,033 ± 458		
MTC	T12, P1	PEC	10:1	2,428 ± 116	38.0[f]	0.010
		PEC	5:1	3,327 ± 416	20.0	
		IT	10:1	3,187 ± 204	16.0	
		IT	5:1	4,125 ± 374	5.0	
		None	0	4,178 ± 374		
MTPa	T12, P1	PEC	10:1	701 ± 33	75.0[f]	0.002
		PEC	5:1	1,032 ± 83	54.0	
		IT	10:1	1,463 ± 550	27.0[f]	
		IT	5:1	2,776 ± 72	0	
		None	0	2,215 ± 180		

[a]   Clonal lines after one passage in vivo at the in vitro passage represented by T-number.

[b]   PEC, thioglycolate-elicited peritoneal macrophages stimulated in vitro with LPS (50 ng/mℓ); IT, intratumoral macrophages isolated from tumors as described in "Materials and Methods", macrophages stimulated in vitro with LPS (50 ng/mℓ).

[c]   Percentage of cytolysis was calculated as

$$\% \text{ of cytolysis} = \left(1 - \frac{a_1}{a_t}\right) \times 100$$

where a_1 is retained cpm in wells with macrophages, and a_t retained cpm in wells with no macrophages.

[d]   Significance between control and experimental samples at the indicated level determined by one way analysis of variance.

[e]   Mean ± SD.

[f]   Significant difference ($p < 0.01$) between metastatic MTLn3, low-metastatic MTLn2 and MTF7, and nonmetastatic MTC and MTPa sublines determined by the Kruskal-Wallis test.

Reproduced with permission from North, S. M., and Nicolson, G. L., *Cancer Res.*, 45, 1453, 1985.

fresh tumor explants in short-term culture were used as the source of tumor cell targets (Table 2). In this system, the most metastatic line (MTLn3) was the least sensitive to macrophage-mediated lysis, whereas the less metastatic lines (MTF7, MTLn2, MTC, and MTPa) were more susceptible to this process. These data suggested that time in culture influences the susceptibility of tumor cells to macrophages, and that established, cultured tumor cell lines may not be the most suitable system for examining macrophage-mediated cytolysis. The source of macrophages used in these assays was

Table 3
EXPERIMENTAL PULMONARY METASTASIS
OF B16 MELANOMA AND UV-2237
FIBROSARCOMA IN 3- AND 10-WEEK-OLD
NUDE MICE[a]

	Median number (range) of lung colonies[b]	
Tumor cells	3-week-old mice	10-week-old mice
B16-F10	98(35—300)[c]	4(0—8)
UV-2237	65(22—110)[c]	0(0—2)
UV-2237-M₁	238(110—300)[c]	1(0—4)
UV-2237-M₂	All 300[c]	2(0—6)

[a] 3- and 8-week-old nude mice were injected intravenously with 30,000 B16-F10 melanoma or 100,000 UV-2237, UV-2237-M₁, and M₂ fibrosarcoma tumor cells.

[b] 20 mice per group. Mice were killed 3 to 4 weeks following tumor inoculation. The lungs were fixed in Bouin's solution and the number of lung colonies was determined with the aid of a dissecting microscope.

[c] The number of lung tumor colonies differed between the age groups ($p < 0.001$), Mann-Whitney U-test.

Reproduced with permission from Hanna, N. *Int. J. Cancer*, 26, 675, 1980.

also important, and our data caused to question the assumption that PECs are a suitable and convenient source of effector cells. To assess the possible functional status of macrophages in vivo it may be necessary to evaluate the activity of intratumoral macrophages and use these effectors in conjunction with their natural target cells isolated from fresh explants of tumors growing *in situ*.

Although enough information has been accumulated to indicate that malignant cells are heterogeneous in their macrophage sensitivities, some authors persist in stating that all tumor cells are equally sensitive to macrophage antitumor mechanisms. Data to support a uniform macrophage sensitivity hypothesis came mainly from two types of negative experiment. First, efforts to sequentially select macrophage-resistant subpopulations were not successful, in contrast to similar selections for T-cell and natural killer (NK)-cell resistant tumor sublines. The reasons for this are not immediately obvious, but they could be related to the source of tumor cells used for such studies, as discussed above. Second, the assays used to demonstrate uniform macrophage sensitivities of tumor cells were usually conducted at such artificially high effector:target cell ratios that differences may not have been observable. Again, the source of cells for such assays may be extremely important.

B. Natural Killer Cells

Another host mechanism important in the destruction of disseminated tumor cells seems to be mediated by NK cells (reviewed in References 99 to 103). Metastatic tumor cells are susceptible to the effects of host surveillance while in the circulation, and Hanna and Fidler[101-103] indicated that this is the point in the metastatic cascade at which NK cells are most effective against malignant cells. Using animals with low NK activity (beige mice) or animals with high NK activity (nude mice), Hanna[103] found that lung colonization correlated with the NK-mediated destruction of tumor cells in the circulation (Table 3). Data obtained from the nude mouse were particularly interesting, because young nude mice (3-weeks-old) have low NK activities, while older mice (older than 6 weeks) have higher NK activities. The difference in NK activity correlates with metastasis in certain tumors. In older nude mice some tumors failed to form experimental metastases, whereas in the young nudes these same tumors displayed a high metastatic potential.

In vitro selection procedures have been used to obtain NK-resistant tumor cell variants. Gorelik et al.[104] and Hanna and Fidler[102] used different animal tumor models and different selection procedures, but both research groups were able to select NK-resistant tumor variant sublines. Assays of these cell sublines in vivo indicated that the selected sublines formed increased numbers of metastases. It appears, therefore, that although many tumors are susceptible to NK-mediated cytolysis, others might not be.

Studies of patients have resulted in little evidence to support the experimental data that NK cells are important in metastasis.[105] NK activities were shown to decline in some patients with substantial tumor burdens,[106] but it has been possible to augment NK responses under conditions designed to increase host immunity. Although there is evidence of a correlation between high NK activity and inhibition of blood-borne metastasis in several animal tumor models, data on the existence of a relationship between NK activity and human cancer metastasis are not convincing.

C. T-Lymphocytes

The original postulate of "immune surveillance" advanced by Burnett[107] suggested that the immune system specifically recognizes TAA, and that tumor cells possessing these determinants could be specifically eradicated by a T-cell-dependent mechanism. But, Moller and Moller[108] demonstrated subsequently that animals deprived of functional T-cells showed neither a greater incidence of spontaneous tumors nor an enhanced susceptibility to tumor induction by carcinogens. In view of this, the concept of immune surveillance fell into disrepute in recent years. Nevertheless, although the original proposal was an admitted oversimplification, there is evidence to substantiate the importance of T-cell-mediated antitumor immunity in a few tumor systems.

To elucidate T-cell-mediated antitumor responses against malignant cells, studies conducted in the early to mid 1970s concentrated on the effects of either lymphocyte depletion on metastasis,[108-111] or on the ability of T-cells to confer antimetastatic protection to naive hosts by the transfer of spleen cells or lymphocyte subpopulations.[112-115] Immune depletion was examined using antilymphocyte serum,[109] neonatal thymectomy and whole-body irradiation,[110] chronic lymph drainage,[111] immunosuppressive drugs, such as cyclosporin A,[116] and the use of congenitally athymic animals.[117] A general consensus from most of these experiments was that T-cell-mediated immunity may be important in preventing metastasis in certain tumor systems. In one series of experiments by Eccles et al.,[117] immunogenic rat fibrosarcomas that were not spontaneously metastatic in the syngeneic host metastasized extensively when transplanted into nude rats.

T-cell antitumor responses may not always be beneficial to the host. T-suppressor cells generated in a "low zone tolerance" response by the presence of slow-growing tumors were shown to be detrimental.[118] Kripke[119] studied immune reactivity of the autochthonous host during ultraviolet light-induced carcinogenesis in mice. Although this system represents one extreme in tumor antigenicity, Kripke and Fisher[120] demonstrated that these highly antigenic tumors were not rejected in animals that were first rendered immunologically deficient. In other experiments, brief intermittent doses of ultraviolet light rendered the recipients tolerant to tumor transplantation, which indicated the occurrence of a specific immune response.[121] This effect was later shown to be caused by the induction or activation of T-suppressor lymphocytes that prevented immune-mediated destruction of the tumor cells.[122] The fact that Fujimoto et al.[123-125]

were able to transfer spleen and thymus cells from tumor-bearing animals further demonstrated the presence of tumor-specific suppressor cells.[125]

In some tumor systems T-cell-resistant variants have been generated that possess altered metastatic properties. For example, Bosslet and Schirrmacher,[126] were able to derive T-cell-resistant variants of the ESb lymphoma isolated from spleen metastases, but not from lung or liver metastases, or from the subcutaneous inoculum site.[127] Schirrmacher and Bosslet[127] were unable to demonstrate the presence of immunoresistant variants in the parental ESb population; they suggested that the immunoresistant variants arose at high frequency, were stable, and possibly generated by a process of specific induction instead of selective enrichment of stable variant subpopulations. Drawing an analogy to parasite immunology,[128,129] Schirrmacher et al.[130] postulated that the microenvironment of the tumor may lead to rapid activation of normally quiescent genetic programs in tumor cells, which results in rapid and stable changes in their malignant phenotypes. The nature of these inductive signals has not been elucidated, but several possibilities have been suggested (see Figure 1, and References 15 and 23).

IV. ANTIBODY-MEDIATED MECHANISMS AGAINST METASTASES

Natural and immune humoral responses to growing and disseminating neoplasms have received less critical attention than cell-mediated antitumor mechanisms. This is probably partly a reflection of the difficulties encountered in quantitating serum antibodies to TAA, and the sensitivities of the assays available. There is some evidence, however, that autologous humoral antitumor responses can occur in humans[131,132] as well as in experimental animals. Gorer[133] was among the first to indicate that antibodies may play a role in allograft rejection, data that stimulated interest in the possible use of antibodies for antitumor immunotherapy.[134-136] Classic investigations using high-titer alloantiserum in transplanted tumor systems demonstrated that tumors of lymphoid origin are more susceptible to the effects of serum antibodies[137] than solid tumors.[138,139]

A. Polyclonal Antibodies

"Natural" antitumor antibodies have been detected in the serum of tumor-bearing animals that are capable of mounting a response that results in the inhibition of metastasis.[140-142] For example, Vaage[141] found that natural serum immune components (antibody plus complement) were able to kill malignant murine mammary carcinoma and ovarian carcinoma cells in vitro and in vivo. Chow et al.[143] examined the levels of natural antitumor antibodies for their importance in tumor surveillance and found that these effects were T-independent. Unfortunately, the mechanism by which "natural" antitumor antibodies mediate their activities was not demonstrated, but it seems likely that these effects are mediated by an antibody-macrophage response.

It is possible that natural responses to syngeneic or autologous tumors reflect cross-reactions between defective cell-surface components possibly glycoproteins, and pre-existing, environmentally induced immunity. For example, the alteration of a single sugar residue in a carbohydrate side-chain can radically alter the antigenicity of a glycoprotein, and it is well known that the antigenic specificities of many human blood group substances, such as the ABH and MN, are determined by oligosaccharides. Minor alterations in the terminal sugars on these oligosaccharide chains influence their antigenicity and immunogenicity. One such example is the Thomsen-Friedenreich antigen or T-antigen.[144] Springer et al.[145] demonstrated the presence of this determinant on the surfaces of breast carcinoma cells, but T-antigen has not been found on benign cells of the breast. Patients with breast cancer have been reported to have low titers of anti-T antibody, presumedly because of its exhaustion by reaction with secreted T-antigen, whose levels return to normal after removal of the primary tumor.[146]

Although antitumor antibodies have been detected in a number of syngeneic systems,[147-151] the therapeutic value of these syngeneic antibodies has not been extensively investigated. In some cases the presence of circulating antibodies to tumor antigens correlated with a poor prognosis and poor host survival.[151] This led to the belief that the efferent arm of the immune system was "blocked" by antibodies combining with antigens, thereby "protecting" tumor cells from immune destruction. The blocking nature of these antibodies was studied by colony inhibition assays in vitro in the absence of added exogenous complement.[152] By definition, such blocking factors present in vivo would be noncomplement-binding because they do not initiate a cytotoxic response. Moller[153] demonstrated that the passive transfer of syngeneic antiserum facilitated the growth of methylcholanthrene-induced mouse sarcomata in the strain of origin and, on the basis of these data, proposed that antibodies may function as "enhancing" factors by altering the apparent immunogenicity of the tumor, thus explaining why antigenic tumors are able to grow and metastasize.[153]

The failure to detect circulating antibodies in many experimental systems, and also in human cancer, may be a result of antibodies complexing with circulating antigens or disseminating tumor cells. Thompson et al.[154] demonstrated the presence of such circulating antigen in the serum of tumor-bearing rats, and other studies demonstrated the existence of antitumor antibody after removal of the primary tumor.[155]

Most of the tumor models investigated for antitumor antibody effects have been solid tumors, such as melanomas,[156,157] fibrosarcomas,[158,159] and carcinomas.[160-162] In such cases, the degree of tumor vascularization and compartmentalization limits the accessibility of tumor cells to blood-borne soluble mediators, such as immunoglobulins. Hence, the relatively small numbers of disseminating cells are most vulnerable to antibody-mediated cellular cytotoxicity (ADCC) or complement-mediated cytolysis. The phenomenon of ADCC has been elegantly demonstrated in vitro,[163] but its relevance in vivo is far from certain. The apparent unimportance of such a mechanism for eradicating neoplastic cells is disappointing; this may be due to the difficulty of establishing in vivo the precise requirements of antigen, antibody, and effector cells in juxtaposition and concentrations suitable to initiate ADCC at levels high enough to substantially influence tumor dissemination.

B. Monoclonal Antibodies

In the subsection above we presented some of the problems of attempting to evaluate the potential importance of antibodies in antitumor responses. However, hybridoma technology[164] has renewed interest, not only in the potential use of monoclonal antibodies (MAb) in tumor detection and antitumor therapy,[165] but also in dissection of the cell surfaces of normal and neoplastic cells in an attempt to understand the nature of host/tumor interactions. The original expectation was that MAb would finally confirm the presence of tumor-specific antigens. This did not happen and, in fact, all recent data suggest that we are unlikely to find tumor-specific antigens. But we learned that antibody specificity can be a function of the screening assays employed rather than a biological phenomenon.

One particularly striking feature revealed by the use of MAb in defining antigen distribution in tumor tissues is the extensive heterogeneity of binding that has been encountered.[166-171] No MAb has yet been shown to yield homogeneous staining of all tumor cells within a single tumor. In a recent review, Edwards[171] drew attention to the fact that most of the MAb generated against cell surface antigens of epithelial cells were directed against carbohydrate specificities.[172-176] Thus, it is pertinent to ask whether tumor heterogeneity is, in part, the consequence of defective protein and glycolipid glycosylation. Structural changes in carbohydrates may lead to functional differences that may be important in metastasis.

Biological studies using passively transferred antitumor MAb have concentrated mostly on leukemias. For example, Bernstein et al.[177] demonstrated that a murine T-cell leukemia could be eradicated by the passive transfer of an anti-Thy 1.1 MAb. The efficacy of MAb treatment is known to depend on the initial tumor cell inoculum and the addition of exogenous complement. Using a murine leukemia model, Kirch and Hammerling[178] found that antibody isotype was important and that, in general, IgG antibodies were more efficient than IgM antibodies.

Clinical studies, such as those of Nadler et al.,[179] Miller et al.,[180] and Ritz et al.,[181] have also concentrated on using MAb against leukemias and lymphomas. Although the patients responded initially to passive MAb infusion, the treatment was not successful, possibly because of "antigenic modulation" or the presence of excessive amounts of free-antigen in the circulation, which can rapidly remove the circulating antibody. The most successful clinical use of MAb was the treatment of a B-cell lymphoma with an MAb directed against the idiotype of the immunoglobulin produced by a specific lymphoma, a truly "tumor-specific" antigen.[182]

Data on the effectiveness of antitumor antibodies in experimental solid tumor systems are scarce. North and Dean[183] were able to demonstrate a significant effect of MAb on the spontaneous metastasis of a rat fibrosarcoma. The MAb was an IgG$_{2b}$ that bound to tumor cells but, within the limits of the assays, did not bind to normal rat tissues.[184] MAb was administered intravenously into syngeneic, congenitally athymic nude rats during the period of tumor growth and after excision of the primary tumor, until the first control rat died. North and Dean's data indicated that the passive transfer of a syngeneic MAb prevented metastatic disease, at least in this system (Table 4). The fact that they were able to use syngeneic nude rats eliminated the involvement of T-cell responsiveness. Although the antitumor mechanism operating in vivo was not determined, circumstantial evidence strongly implicated host effector cells, because sera and plasma alone (containing high titers of the MAb) were not cytotoxic when tested in vitro. Herlyn and Koprowski[185] have presented circumstantial evidence that implicated the macrophage in antibody-mediated inhibition of growth of human xenografts in nude mice.

An interesting aspect of the preliminary work by North and Dean[183] was the total eradication of metastases in about one half of the treated animals, with a concurrent enhancement of metastatic growth in the remainder. These researchers proposed that this may reflect a heterogeneity in the tumor cell population or in antigen density on the tumor cells. They also noted a similar phenomenon when cells were injected intravenously in the presence of MAb. Elimination or enhancement of tumor growth seemed to be related to the concentration of the MAb administered and to the time after injection of tumor cells that antibody was given. The data suggested that effector cells might be involved with the MAb mechanism and that an active immune response occurred to the passively transferred antibody.

The network hypothesis of immune regulation advanced by Jerne[186] anticipated the presence of a negative feedback mechanism to control the immune response to an antigenic stimulus. In general, a tumor growing in the autochthonous host grows slowly, with a cell-doubling time of months. The slow growth of such a tumor, with sparsely situated potential tumor antigens, may induce a "low zone tolerance" to the tumor. Induction of tolerance to the tumor may result in immune dysfunction, a possible consequence of which could be the generation of anti-idiotypic antibodies or anti-idiotypic T-suppressor cells. Anti-immunoglobulins can be generated against the Fc portion (rheumatoid factors) of the immunoglobulin molecule[187,188] or against the Fab variable (anti-idiotype) region.[189] Studies of human melanoma showed the presence of

Table 4

EFFECT OF PASSIVELY TRANSFERRED ANTIBODY ON THE METASTASIS OF MC24 FIBROSARCOMA IN NUDE RATS

Experiment No.	Treatment	No. lung tumor colonies	Lung weights (g)	Time of death[a] (days post amputation)
1	PBS[b]	>200,>200,>200,	2.0,2.0,2.0,	59,61,73
		>200,>200	2.5,2.6	73,73
	M10/76[c]	0,6,50,>200,	(1.3,1.6,1.6,ND)[e]	73,73,73,70,
		>200,>200,>200,>200	(9.8,8.0,8.7,6.2)[e]	73,73,73,73
	11/160[d]	150,>200,>200,ND	1.9,ND,ND,1.9,	63,70,70,73
		>200,>200,>200,>200	2.1,3.4,2.4,5.9	73,73,73,73
2	PBS	>200,>200,>200,>200,>200,>200	ND,ND,8.0,5.6,3.6,3.9,	49,53,60,60,60,60
		>200,>200,>200,>200,>200	6.3,4.1,5.0,5.5,10.7	60,60,60,60,60
	M10/76	7,8,8,11,12,13,22,	(2.1,2.3,2.4,2.9,2.7,2.12.6)[e]	60,60,60,60,60,60,60,
		>200,>200,>200,>200,>200	(6.6,8.9,6.7,8.4,10.1)[e]	60,55,58,58,60
	11/160	>200,>200,>200,>200,>200	3.0,3.4,5.9,6.1,7.3,	60,60,60,60,60,
		>200,>200,>200,>200	8.1,8.2,8.5, 9.2	60,60,60,60,

[a] Experiment 1 was terminated 73 days after amputation of the tumor, at this time all surviving rats were killed. Experiment 2 was terminated 60 days after amputation. For experimental details see reference number 183.

[b] Abbreviations: PBS; phosphate buffered saline ND; not determined.

[c] M10/76 is a rat IgG$_{2b}$ MAb with specificity for the MC24 fibrosarcoma.[184]

[d] 11/160 is a rat IgG$_{2b}$ MAb which does not react with the MC24 fibrosarcoma.[184]

[e] Significant difference ($p < 0.005$) between treated groups and normal controls determined by student t-test.

anti-idiotypic antibody and immune complexes in the serum of patients with malignant melanoma.[190] All patients with disseminated disease had immune complexes, whereas only 18% of patients with localized disease had detectable immune complexes. It is well known from disease states other than malignancy that immune complexes are significant in the immune regulation of the disease state, and they may, therefore, possibly influence tumor metastasis.[190]

It is apparent from recent studies that humoral responses to tumor antigens can occur in humans.[191] Schlom and co-workers used lymph node cells from a mastectomy patient to produce an MAb with specificity for a breast tumor-associated antigen.[191] Whether this MAb has biological activity remains to be determined. When considering the effectiveness of the humoral immune response to tumors, immunoglobulin isotype may be of considerable importance in evaluating the antibody's potential biological activity.[192,193] Not only do the different immunoglobulin isotypes have different effector functions, they also recognize distinct biochemical entities.[194-201]

V. CONCLUDING COMMENT

Tumor metastasis is a complex process that involves both tumor and host properties. In this brief introduction of the various parameters of the immune system that may be relevant to metastasis, we have probably not demonstrated forcefully enough the complexity of the problems faced by both basic investigators and the clinicians, in understanding and ultimately treating metastatic disease. Although no perfect experimental tumor system is available to study host effects on metastasis, valuable information about the nature of host antitumor reactivity will be acquired. Once we have fuller knowledge of the regulatory mechanisms operative during tumor/host interactions, we will be able to evaluate the importance of host mechanisms in metastatic disease.

REFERENCES

1. Fidler, I. J. and Hart, I. R., Biological diversity in metastatic neoplasms. Origins and implications, *Science,* 217, 998, 1982.
2. Hart, I. R. and Fidler, I. J., The implications of tumor heterogeneity for studies of the biology and therapy of cancer metastasis, *Biochim. Biophys. Acta,* 651, 37, 1981.
3. Nicolson, G. L., Cancer metastasis: organ colonization and the cell surface properties of malignant cells, *Biochim. Biophys. Acta,* 695, 113, 1982.
4. Nicolson, G. L. and Poste, G., Tumor cell diversity and host responses in cancer metastasis. I. Properties of metastatic cells, *Curr. Probl. Cancer,* 7(6), 1, 1982.
5. Nicolson, G. L. and Poste, G., Tumor cell diversity and host responses in cancer metastasis. II. Host immune responses and therapy of metastases, *Curr. Probl. Cancer,* 7(7), 1, 1983.
6. Heppner, G. H., Tumor heterogeneity, *Cancer Res.,* 44, 2259, 1984.
7. Griffin, J. E., Allman, D. R., Durrant, J. L., and Wilson, J. D., Variation in steroid 5-reductase activity in cloned skin fibroblasts, *J. Biol. Chem.,* 256, 3662, 1981.
8. Peterson, J. A., Bartholomew, J. C., Stampfer, M., and Ceriani, R. L., Analysis of expression of human mammary epithelial antigens in normal and malignant breast cells at the single cell level by flow cytofluorimetry, *Exp. Cell. Biol.,* 49, 1, 1981.
9. Peterson, J. A., Ceriani, R. L., Blank, E. W., and Osvaldo, L., Comparison of rates of phenotypic variability in surface antigen expression in normal and cancerous breast epithelial cells, *Cancer Res.,* 43, 4291, 1983.
10. Foulds, L., The histologic analysis of mammary tumors in mice. I. Scope of investigations and general principles of analysis, *J. Natl. Cancer Inst.,* 17, 701, 1956.
11. Foulds, L., The histologic analysis of mammary tumors in mice. II. The histology of responsiveness and progression. The origin of tumors, *J. Natl. Cancer Inst.,* 17, 713, 1956.
12. Foulds, L., *Neoplastic Development,* Academic Press, New York, 1975.
13. Nowell, P. C., The clonal evolution of tumor cell populations, *Science,* 194, 23, 1976.
14. Nowell, P. C., Tumor progression and clonal evolution. The role of genetic instability, in *Chromosome mutation and neoplasia,* German, J., Ed., Alan R. Liss, New York, 1983, 413.
15. Nicolson, G. L., Tumor progression, oncogenes and the evolution of metastatic phenotypic diversity, *Clin. Exp. Met.,* 2, 85, 1984.
16. Wolman, S. R., Karyotypic progression in human tumors, *Cancer Met. Rev.,* 2, 257, 1983.
17. Cifone, M. A. and Fidler, I. J., Increasing metastatic potential is associated with increasing genetic instability of clones isolated from murine neoplasms, *Proc. Natl. Acad. Sci. U.S.A.,* 78, 6949, 1981.
18. Bosslet, K. and Schirrmacher, V., High-frequency generation of new immunoresistant tumor variants during metastasis of a cloned murine tumor line (Esb), *Int. J. Cancer,* 29, 195, 1982.
19. Chow, D. A. and Greenberg, A. H., The generation of tumor heterogeneity *in vivo, Int. J. Cancer,* 25, 261, 1980.
20. Stackpole, C. W., Generation of phenotypic diversity in the B16 mouse melanoma relative to spontaneous metastasis, *Cancer Res.,* 43, 3057, 1983.
21. Dennis, J. W., Donaghue, T. P., and Kerbel, R. S., An examination of tumor antigen loss in spontaneous metastasis, *Invasion Met.,* 1, 111, 1981.
22. Neri, A. and Nicolson, G. L., Phenotypic drift of metastatic and cell surface properties of mammary adenocarcinoma cell clones, *Int. J. Cancer,* 28, 731, 1981.
23. Nicolson, G. L., Generation of phenotypic diversity and progression in metastatic tumors, *Cancer Met. Rev.,* 3, 25, 1984.
24. Nicolson, G. L., Cell surface molecules and tumor metastasis. Regulation of metastatic diversity, *Exp. Cell Res.,* 150, 3, 1984.
25. Heppner, G. H., The challenge of tumor heterogeneity, in *Commentaries on Research in Breast Disease,* Vol. 1, Bulbrook and Taylor, Eds., Alan R. Liss, New York, 1979, 177.
26. Owens, A. H., Jr., Coffey, D. S., and Baylin, S. B., *Tumor Cell Heterogeneity: Origins and Implications,* Academic Press, New York, 1982.
27. Kerbel, R. S., Dennis, J. W., Largarde, A. E., and Frost, P., Tumor progression in metastasis: an experimental approach using lectin resistant tumor variants, *Cancer Met. Rev.,* 1, 99, 1982.
28. Neri, A., Welch, D. R., Kawaguchi, T., and Nicolson, G. L., The development and biologic properties of malignant cell sublines and clones of a spontaneously metastasizing rat mammary adenocarcinoma, *J. Natl. Cancer Inst.,* 68, 507, 1982.
29. Poste, G., Doll, J., and Fidler, I. J., Interactions among clonal subpopulations affect stability of the metastatic phenotype in polyclonal populations of B16 melanoma cells, *Proc. Natl. Acad. Sci. U.S.A.,* 78, 6226, 1981.

30. Reading, C. L., Belloni, P. N., and Nicolson, G. L., Selection and *in vivo* properties of lectin attachment variants of malignant murine lymphosarcoma cell lines, *J. Natl. Cancer Inst.*, 64, 1241, 1980.

31. Kripke, M. L., Gruys, E., and Fidler, I. J., Metastatic heterogeneity of cells from an ultraviolet light-induced murine fibrosarcoma of recent origin, *Cancer Res.*, 38, 2962, 1978.

32. Frost, P. and Kerbel, R. S., Immunoselection *in vitro* of a non-metastatic variant from a highly metastatic tumor, *Int. J. Cancer*, 27, 381, 1981.

33. Frost, P. and Kerbel, R. S., On the possible epigenetic mechanism(s) of tumor cell heterogeneity, *Cancer Met. Rev.*, 2, 375, 1983.

34. Schirrmacher, V., Shifts in tumor cell phenotypes induced by signals from the microenvironment: relevance for immunobiology of cancer metastasis, *Immunobiology*, 157, 89, 1980.

35. Bissell, M. J., Hall, H. G., and Parry, G., How does the extracellular matrix direct gene expression, *J. Theor. Biol.*, 99, 31, 1983.

36. Mintz, G. and Illmense, K., Normal genetically mosaic mice produced from malignant teratocarcinoma cells, *Proc. Natl. Acad. Sci. U.S.A.*, 72, 3585, 1975.

37. Sachs, L., Constitutive uncoupling of pathways of gene expression that control growth and differentiation in myeloid leukemia: a model for the origin and progression of malignancy, *Proc. Natl. Acad. Sci. U.S.A.*, 77, 6152, 1980.

38. Fidler, I. J. and Nicolson, G. L., Immunobiology of experimental metastatic melanoma, *Cancer Biol. Rev.*, 2, 171, 1981.

39. Ioachim, H. L., Keller, S. E., Dorsett, B. H., and Pearse, A., Induction of partial immunologic tolerance in rats and progressive loss of cellular antigenicity in gross virus leukemia, *J. Exp. Med.*, 139, 1382, 1984.

40. Stutman, O., Immunodepression and malignancy, *Adv. Cancer Res.*, 22, 261, 1975.

41. Eccles, S. A. and Alexander, P., Immunologically mediated restraint of latent tumor metastasis, *Nature (London)*, 257, 52, 1975.

42. Davey, G. C., Currie, G. A., and Alexander, P., Immunity as the predominant factor determining metastasis of murine lymphoma, *Br. J. Cancer*, 40, 590, 1979.

43. Hewitt, H. B., The choice of animal tumors for experimental studies of cancer therapy, *Adv. Cancer Res.*, 27, 149, 1978.

44. Hewitt, H. B., A critical examination of the foundations of immunotherapy for cancer, *Clin. Radiol.*, 30, 361, 1979.

45. Baldwin, R. W., Immunological aspects of chemical carcinogenesis, *Adv. Cancer Res.*, 18, 1, 1973.

46. Natori, T., Law, L. W., and Appella, E., Immunochemical evidence of a tumor-specific surface antigen obtained by detergent solubilization of the membranes of a chemically induced sarcoma, Meth-A, *Cancer Res.*, 38, 359, 1978.

47. Bauer, H., Virion and tumor cell antigens of C-type RNA tumor viruses, *Adv. Cancer Res.*, 20, 275, 1975.

48. Attia, A. M. and Weiss, W., Immunology of spontaneous mammary carcinomas in mice (v). Acquired tumor resistance and enhancement in strain A mice infected with mammary tumor virus, *Cancer Res.*, 26, 1787, 1966.

49. Alexander, P., Dormant metastases which manifest on immunosuppression and the role of macrophages in tumors, in *Fundamental Aspects of Metastasis*, Weiss, L., Ed., North-Holland, Amsterdam, 1976, 227.

50. Wheelock, E. F., Weinhold, K. J., and Lerich, J., The tumor dormant state, *Adv. Cancer Res.*, 34, 107, 1981.

51. Woodruff, M. F. A., Interaction of cancer and host, *Br. J. Cancer*, 46, 313, 1982.

52. Prehn, R. T., The immune reactions as a stimulator of tumor growth, *Science*, 176, 170, 1972.

53. Prehn, R. T., Do tumors grow because of the immune response of the host?, *Transplant. Rev.*, 28, 34, 1976.

54. Umiel, T. and Trainin, N., Immunological enhancement of tumor growth by syngeneic thymus derived lymphocytes, *Transplantation*, 18, 244, 1974.

55. Small, M. and Trainin, N., Separation of populations of sensitized lymphoid cells into fractions inhibiting and fractions enhancing syngeneic tumor growth *in vivo*, *J. Immunol.*, 117, 292, 1976.

56. Sugarbaker, E. V. and Cohen, A. M., Altered antigenicity in spontaneous pulmonary metastases from an antigenic murine sarcoma, *Surgery*, 72, 155, 1972.

57. Pimm, M. V. and Baldwin, R. W., Antigenic differences between primary methylcholanthrene-induced rat sarcomas and post-surgical recurrences, *Int. J. Cancer*, 20, 37, 1977.

58. Fogel, M., Gorelik, E., Segal, S., and Feldman, M., Differences in cell surface antigens of tumor metastases and those of the local tumor, *J. Natl. Cancer Inst.*, 62, 585, 1979.

59. Calabresi, P., Dexter, D. L., and Heppner, G. H., Clinical and pharmacological implications of cancer cell differentiation and heterogeneity, *Biochem. Pharmacol.*, 28, 1933, 1979.

60. Kim, U., Metastasizing mammary carcinomas in rats: induction and study of their immunogenicity, *Science,* 164, 72, 1970.
61. Dennis, J. W., Donaghue, T. P., and Kerbel, R. S., An examination of tumor antigen loss in spontaneous metastasis, *Invasion Met.,* 1, 111, 1981.
62. Shearman, P. J., Gallatin, W. M., and Longenecker, B. M., Detection of cell surface antigen correlated with organ-specific metastasis, *Nature (London),* 286, 267, 1980.
63. Hanna, M. G., Jr. and Key, M. E., Immunotherapy of metastasis enhances subsequent chemotherapy, *Science,* 217, 367, 1982.
64. Reading, C. L., Brunson, K. W., Torriani, M., and Nicolson, G. L., Malignancies of metastatic murine lymphosarcoma cell lines and clones correlate with decreased cell surface display of RNA tumor virus envelope glycoprotein gp70, *Proc. Natl. Acad. Sci. U.S.A.,* 77, 5943, 1980.
65. Rees, R. C., Shah, L. P., and Baldwin, R. W., Inhibition of pulmonary tumour development in rats sensitized to rat embryonic tissue, *Nature (London),* 255, 329, 1975.
66. Nicolson, G. L., Mascali, J. J., and McGuire, E. J., Metastatic RAW117 lymphosarcoma as a model for malignant-normal cell interactions. Possible roles for cell surface antigens in determining the quantity and location of secondary tumors, *Oncodevelop. Biol. Med.,* 4, 149, 1982.
67. Reading, C. L., Kraemer, P. M., Miner, K. M., and Nicolson, G. L., *In vivo* and *in vitro* properties of malignant variants of RAW117 metastatic murine lymphoma/lymphosarcoma, *Clin. Exp. Met.,* 1, 125, 1983.
68. Currie, G. A. and Basham, C., Serum-mediated inhibition of the immunological reactions of the patient to his own tumor, *Br. J. Cancer,* 26, 472, 1972.
69. Berry, N., Jones, D. B., Smallwood, J., Taylor, I., Kirkham, N., and Taylor-Papadimitriou, J., The prognostic value of the monoclonal antibodies HMFG-1 and HMGF-2 in breast cancer, *Br. J. Cancer,* 51, 179, 1985.
70. Neri, A., Ruoslahti, E., and Nicolson, G. L., The distribution of fibronectin in clonal cell lines of a rat mammary adenocarcinoma growing *in vitro* and *in vivo* at primary and metastatic sites, *Cancer Res.,* 41, 5082, 1981.
71. Welch, D. R., Milas, L., Tomasovic, S. P., and Nicolson, G. L., Heterogeneous response and clonal drift of sensitivities of metastatic 13762NF mammary adenocarcinoma clones to gamma radiation *in vitro, Cancer Res.,* 43, 6, 1983.
72. Welch, D. R. and Nicolson, G. L., Phenotypic drift and heterogeneity in response of metastatic mammary adenocarcinoma cell clones to Adriamycin, 5-fluoro-2′-deoxyuridine, and methotrexate treatment *in vitro, Clin. Exp. Met.,* 1, 319, 1983.
73. Steck, P. A. and Nicolson, G. L., Cell surface glycoproteins of 13762NF mammary adenocarcinoma clones of differing metastatic potentials, *Exp. Cell Res.,* 147, 265, 1983.
74. North, S. M. and Nicolson, G. L., Effect of host immune status on the spontaneous metastasis of cloned cell lines of the 13762NF rat mammary adenocarcinoma, *Br. J. Cancer,* 57, 747, 1985.
75. Alexander, P., Surveillance against neoplastic cells: is it mediated by macrophage?, *Br. J. Cancer,* 33, 344, 1976.
76. Alexander, P., Metastatic spread and "escape" from the immune defenses of the host, *Natl. Cancer Inst. Monogr.,* 44, 125, 1976.
77. Nelson, D. S., Non-specific immunoregulation by macrophages and their products, in *Immunobiology of the Macrophages,* Nelson, D. S., Ed., Academic Press, New York, 1976, 235.
78. Eccles, S. A. and Alexander, P., Macrophage content of tumours in relation to metastatic spread and host immune reaction, *Nature (London),* 250, 667, 1974.
79. Eccles, S. A. and Alexander, P., Sequestration of macrophages in growing tumors and its effect on the immunological capacity of the host, *Br. J. Cancer,* 30, 22, 1974.
80. Birbeck, M. S. and Carter, R. L., Observations on the ultrastructure of two hamster lymphomas with particular reference to infiltrating macrophages, *Int. J. Cancer,* 9, 249, 1972.
81. Wood, G. W. and Gillespie, G. Y., Studies on the role of macrophages in regulation of growth and metastasis of murine chemically induced fibrosarcoma, *Int. J. Cancer,* 16, 1022, 1975.
82. Evans, R. and Lawler, E. M., Macrophage content and immunogenicity of C57BL/6J and BALB/cBYJ methylcholanthrene induced sarcomas, *Int. J. Cancer,* 26, 831, 1980.
83. Talmadge, J. E., Key, M., and Fidler, I. J., Macrophage content of metastatic and non-metastatic rodent neoplasms, *J. Immunol.,* 126, 2245, 1981.
84. Mahoney, K. H. and Heppner, G. H., Tumor associated macrophages of mouse mammary tumors. II. Differential distribution of macrophages from metastatic and non-metastatic tumors, *J. Immunol.,* 131, 2079, 1983.
85. Vose, B. M., Cytotoxicity of adherent cells associated with some human tumors and lung tissues, *Cancer Immunol. Immunother.,* 5, 173, 1978.
86. Gauci, C. L. and Alexander, P., The macrophage content of some human tumors, *Cancer Lett.,* 1, 29, 1975.

87. Alexander, P., Eccles, S. A., and Gauci, C. L., The significance of macrophages in human and experimental tumors, *Ann. N.Y. Acad. Sci.,* 276, 124, 1976.

88. Shin, H. S., Economou, J. S., Pasternack, G. R., Johnson, R. J., and Hayden, M. L., Antibody mediated suppression of grafted lymphoma, *J. Exp. Med.,* 144, 1274, 1976.

89. Haskill, J. S., Key, M. E., Rador, L. A., Parthenais, E., Karn, J. H., Fett, J. W., Yamamura, Y., Delustro, F., Vesley, J., and Gant, G., The importance of antibody and macrophages in spontaneous and drug-mediated regression of T1699 mammary adenocarcinoma, *J. Reticuendothelial Soc.,* 26, 417, 1979.

90. Evans, R. and Alexander, P., Mechanism of immunologically specific killing of tumour cells by macrophages, *Nature (London),* 236, 168, 1972.

91. Wiltrout, R. H., Brunda, M. J., and Holden, H. T., Variation in selectivity of tumor cell cytolysis by murine macrophages, macrophage-like cell lines and NK cells, *Int. J. Cancer,* 30, 335, 1982.

92. Pross, H. F. and Kerbel, R. S., An assessment of intra-tumor phagocytic and surface marker-bearing cells in a series of autochthonous and early passaged chemically induced murine sarcomas, *J. Natl. Cancer Inst.,* 57, 1157, 1976.

93. Miner, K. M., Klostergaard, J., Granger, G., and Nicolson, G. L., Differences in cytotoxic effects of activated murine peritoneal macrophages and J774 monocyte cells on metastatic variants of B16 melanoma, *J. Natl. Cancer Inst.,* 68, 507, 1983.

94. Miner, K. M. and Nicolson, G. L., Differences in the sensitivities of murine metastatic lymphoma/lymphosarcoma variants to macrophage mediated cytolysis and/or cytostasis, *Cancer Res.,* 43, 2063, 1983.

95. Urban, J. L. and Schreiber, H., Selection of macrophage-resistant progressor tumor variants by the normal host, *J. Exp. Med.,* 157, 642, 1983.

96. North, S. M. and Nicolson, G. L., Heterogeneity in the sensitivities of the 13762NF rat mammary adenocarcinoma cell clones to cytolysis mediated by extra- and intratumoral macrophages, *Cancer Res.,* 45, 1453, 1985.

97. Mantovani, A., *In vitro* effects on tumor cells of macrophages isolated from an early passage chemically induced murine sarcoma and from its spontaneous metastases, *Int. J. Cancer,* 27, 221, 1981.

98. Yamamura, Y., Fischer, B. C., Harnaha, J. B., and Proctor, J. W., Heterogeneity of murine mammary adenocarcinoma cell subpopulations. *In vitro* and *in vivo* resistance to macrophage cytotoxicity and its association with metastatic capacity, *Int. J. Cancer,* 33, 67, 1984.

99. Herberman, R. B., Ed., *Natural Cell-Mediated Immunity Against Tumors,* Academic Press, New York, 1980.

100. Herberman, R. B. and Holden, J., Natural cell mediated immunity, *Adv. Cancer Res.,* 7, 305, 1978.

101. Hanna, N. and Fidler, I. J., Role of natural killer cells in the destruction of circulating tumor emboli, *J. Natl. Cancer Inst.,* 65, 801, 1980.

102. Hanna, N. and Fidler, I. J., Relationship between metastatic potential and resistance to natural killer cell-mediated cytotoxicity in three murine tumor systems, *J. Natl. Cancer Inst.,* 66, 1183, 1981.

103. Hanna, N., Expression of metastatic potential of tumor cells in young nude mice is correlated with low levels of natural killer cell-mediated cytotoxicity, *Int. J. Cancer,* 26, 675, 1980.

104. Gorelik, E., Fogel, M., Feldman, M., and Segal, S., Differences in resistance of metastatic tumor cells and cells from local tumor growth to cytotoxicity of natural killer cells, *J. Natl. Cancer Inst.,* 63, 1397, 1979.

105. Golub, S. H., *In situ, in vitro* and systemic regulation of NK cytotoxicity, in *Fundamental Mechanisms in Human Cancer Immunology,* Saunders, J. P., Daniels, J. C., and Serrou, B., Eds., Elsevier/North-Holland, Amsterdam, 1981, 477.

106. Takasugi, M., Ramzeyer, A., and Takasuki, J., Decline of natural non-selective cell-mediated cytotoxicity in patients with tumor progression, *Cancer Res.,* 37, 413, 1977.

107. Burnett, F. M., Immunological surveillance against neoplasm, *Transplant. Rev.,* 7, 3, 1971.

108. Moller, G. and Moller, E., Experiments on the concept of immunological surveillance, *Transplantation Rev.,* 28, 1, 1976.

109. Wagner, J. L. and Haughton, G., Immunosuppression by antilymphocyte serum and its effect on tumors induced by 3-methylcholanthrene, *J. Natl. Cancer Inst.,* 46, 1, 1971.

110. Woodruff, M. F. A., Dumber, N., and Ghaffar, A., The growth of tumours in T-cell deprived mice and their response to treatment with corynebacterium parvum, *Proc. Roy. Soc. Lond. (Biol.),* 184, 97, 1973.

111. Proctor, J. W., Rudenstam, C. M., and Alexander, P., A factor preventing the development of lung metastases in rats with sarcomas, *Nature (London),* 242, 29, 1973.

112. Bhan, A. K., Perry, L. L., Cantor, H., McCluskey, R. T., Bennacerraf, B., and Greene, M. I., The role of T-cell sets in the rejection of a methylcholanthrene-induced sarcoma (S1509a) in syngeneic mice, *Am. J. Pathol.,* 102, 20, 1981.

113. Deckers, P. J., Edgerton, B. W., Thomas, B. S., and Pilch, Y. H., The adoptive transfer of concomitant immunity to murine tumor isografts with spleen cells from tumor bearing animals, *Cancer Res.,* 31, 734, 1971.
114. Gorelik, E., Fogel, M., De Baetselier, P., Katsar, S., Feldman, M., and Segal, S., Immunobiological diversity of metastatic cells, in *Tumor Invasion and Metastasis,* Liotta, L. and Hart, I., Eds., Martinus Nijhoff, Hingham, Mass., 1982, 133.
115. Rosenberg, S. A., Eberlein, T. J., Grimm, E. A., Lotze, M. T., Mazunder, A., and Rosenstein, M., Development of long-term cell lines and lymphoid clones reactive against murine and human tumors: a new approach to the adoptive immunotherapy of cancer, *Surgery,* 92, 328, 1982.
116. Eccles, S. A., Heckford, S. E., and Alexander, P., Effect of cyclosporin on the growth and spontaneous metastasis of syngeneic animal tumours, *Br. J. Cancer,* 42, 252, 1980.
117. Eccles, S. A., Styles, J. M., Hobbs, S. M., and Dean, C. J., Metastasis in the nude rat associated with lack of immune response, *Br. J. Cancer,* 40, 802, 1979.
118. Maier, T. and Levy, J. G., Anti-tumor effects of an antiserum raised in syngeneic mice to a tumor-specific T-suppressor factor, *Cancer Immunol. Immunother.,* 13, 134, 1982.
119. Kripke, M. L., Antigenicity of murine skin tumors induced by ultraviolet light, *J. Natl. Cancer Inst.,* 53, 1333, 1974.
120. Kripke, M. L. and Fisher, M. S., Immunologic parameters of ultraviolet carcinogenesis, *J. Natl. Cancer Inst.,* 57, 211, 1976.
121. Fisher, M. S. and Kripke, M. L., Systemic alteration induced in mice by ultraviolet light irradiation and its relationship to ultraviolet carcinogenesis, *Proc. Natl. Acad. Sci. U.S.A.,* 74, 1668, 1977.
122. Fisher, M. S. and Kripke, M. L., Further studies on the tumor specific suppressor cells induced by ultraviolet light radiation, *J. Immunol.,* 121, 1139, 1978.
123. Fujimoto, S., Green, M., and Sehan, A. H., Immunosuppressor T cells in tumor bearing hosts, *Immunol. Commun.,* 4, 201, 1975.
124. Fujimoto, S., Green, M., and Sehan, A. H., Regulation of the immune response to tumor antigens. I. Immunosuppressor cells in tumor bearing host, *J. Immunol.,* 116, 791, 1976.
125. Fujimoto, S., Matsuzawa, T., Kakagawa, K., and Tada, T., Cellular interaction between cytotoxic and suppressor T cells against syngeneic tumors in the mouse, *Cell. Immunol.,* 38, 378, 1978.
126. Bosslet, K. and Schirrmacher, V., Escape of metastasizing clonal tumor cell variants from tumor-specific cytolytic T-lymphocytes, *J. Exp. Med.,* 154, 557, 1981.
127. Schirrmacher, V. and Bosslet, K., Tumor metastasis and cell mediated immunity in a model system in DBA/2 mice. Immunoselection of tumor variants differing in tumor antigen expression and metastatic capacity, *Int. J. Cancer,* 25, 781, 1979.
128. Vickerman, K., Antigenic variation in trypanosomes, *Nature (London),* 273, 613, 1978.
129. Hoeijmakers, I. H. J., Frasch, A. C. C., Bernard, A., Barst, P., and Cross, G. A. M., Novel expression-linked copies of the genes for various surface antigens in trypanosomes, *Nature (London),* 284, 78, 1980.
130. Schirrmacher, V., Fogel, M., Russmann, E., Bosslet, K., Altevogt, P., and Beck, L., Antigenic variation in cancer metastasis: immune escape versus immune control, *Cancer Met. Rev.,* 1, 241, 1982.
131. Lewis, M. G., Phillips, T. M., and Rowden, G., Serological identification of tumor antigens in human malignant melanoma, in *Serologic Analysis of Human Cancer Antigens,* Academic Press, New York, 1980, 385.
132. Roth, J. A. and Wesley, R. A., Human tumor-associated antigens detected by serologic techniques: analysis of autologous humoral immune responses to primary and metastatic human sarcomas by an enzyme-linked immunoabsorbent solid-phase assay (ELISA), *Cancer Res.,* 42, 3978, 1982.
133. Gorer, P. A., The role of antibodies in immunity to transplanted leukemia in mice, *J. Pathol.,* 54, 51, 1942.
134. De Waal, R. M. W., Cornelissen, I. M. H. A., Capel, P. J. A., and Koene, R. A. P., Passive enhancement of mouse tumor allografts by alloantibodies is Fc-dependent, *J. Immunol.,* 123, 1353, 1979.
135. Lanier, L. L., Babcock, G. F., Raybourne, R. B., Arnold, L. W., Warner, N. L., and Haughton, G., Mechanim of B cell lymphoma immunotherapy with passive xenogeneic anti-idiotype serum, *J. Immunol.,* 125, 1730, 1980.
136. Greene, M. I., Dorf, M. E., Pierres, M., and Benacerraf, B., Reduction of a syngeneic tumor growth by an anti-I-J alloantiserum, *Proc. Natl. Acad. Sci. U.S.A.,* 74, 5118, 1977.
137. Gorer, P. A. and Amos, D. B., Passive immunity in mice against a C57BL leukosis EL4 by means of iso-immune serum, *Cancer Res.,* 16, 338, 1956.
138. Kaliss, N., Immunological enhancement of tumor homografts: a review, *Cancer Res.,* 18, 962, 1958.
139. Gorer, P. A. and Kaliss, N., The effect of isoantibodies *in vivo* on three different transplantable neoplasms in mice, *Cancer Res.,* 19, 824, 1959.

140. Vaage, J., Humoral and cellular immune factors in the systemic control of artificially induced metastases in C3Hf mice, *Cancer Res.*, 1957, 33, 1973.

141. Vaage, J., *In vivo* and *in vitro* lysis of mouse cancer cells by antimetastatic effectors in normal plasma, *Cancer Immunol. Immunother.*, 4, 257, 1978.

142. Vaage, J. and Agrawal, S., Stimulation or inhibition of immune resistance against metastatic or local growth of a C3H mammary carcinoma, *Cancer Res.*, 36, 1831, 1976.

143. Chow, D. A., Wolosin, L. B., and Greenberg, A. H., Murine natural anti-tumor antibodies. II. The contribution of natural antibodies to tumour surveillance, *Int. J. Cancer*, 27, 459, 1981.

144. Friedenreich, V., *The Thomsen Hemagglutination Phenomenon*, Levin and Munksgaard, Copenhagen, 1930.

145. Springer, G. F., Desai, P. R., and Banatwala, I., Blood group MN antigens and precursors in normal and malignant human breast glandular tissue, *Int. J. Cancer*, 54, 335, 1975.

146. Springer, G. F., Murphy, S. M., Desai, P. R., Wurtz, K., Black, S., and Scanlon, E. F., Diagnosis of breast carcinoma with Thomsen-Friedenreich (T) antigen and human anti-T antibody, *Breast*, 7, 24, 1981.

147. Thompson, D. M. P., Eccles, S. A., and Alexander, P., Antibodies and soluble tumor-specific antigens in blood and lymph of rats with chemically induced sarcomata, *Br. J. Cancer*, 28, 6, 1973.

148. Lando, P., Gabriel, J., Berzins, K., and Perlman, P., Determination of the immunoglobulin class of complement-dependent cytotoxic antibodies in serum of D23 hepatoma bearing rats, *Scand. J. Immunol.*, 11, 253, 1980.

149. Gyure, L. A., Dean, C. J., Hall, J. G., and Styles, J. M., Tumor-specific antibodies of the IgA class in rats after the implantation of a syngeneic tumour in the bile of rats, *Int. Arch. Allergy Appl. Immunol.*, 59, 75, 1980.

150. Dean, C. J., Hobbs, S. M., Hopkins, J. U., North, S. M., and Styles, J. M., Syngeneic antitumour antibodies in rats: clearance of cell bound antibody *in vivo* and *in vitro*, *Br. J. Cancer*, 46, 190, 1982.

151. Moller, G., Studies on the mechanism of immunological enhancement of tumor homografts. III. Interactions between humoral isoantibodies and immune lymphoid cells, *J. Natl. Cancer Inst.*, 30, 1205, 1963.

152. Hellstrom, I., Sjogren, H. O., Warner, G., and Hellstrom, K. E., Blocking of cell mediated immunity by sera from patients with growing neoplasms, *Int. J. Cancer*, 7, 226, 1971.

153. Moller, G., Effect on tumour growth in syngeneic recipients of antibodies against tumour-specific antigens in methylcholanthrene-induced mouse sarcomas, *Nature (London)*, 204, 846, 1964.

154. Thompson, D. M. P., Steele, K., and Alexander, P., The presence of tumour-specific membrane antigen in the serum of rats with chemically induced sarcomata, *Br. J. Cancer*, 28, 27, 1973.

155. Baldwin, R. W. and Barker, C. R., Demonstration of tumor specific humoral antibody against aminoazo dye induced hepatoma, *Br. J. Cancer*, 21, 793, 1967.

156. Baniyash, M., Smorodinsky, W. I., Yaakubovicz, M., and Wotz, I. P., Serologically detected MHC and tumor-associated antigens on the B16 melanoma variants and humoral immunity in mice bearing these tumors, *J. Immunol.*, 129, 1318, 1982.

157. Thistlewaithe, P., Davidson, D. D., Fidler, I. J., and Roth, J. A., Syngeneic humoral immune responses to tumor-associated antigens expressed by K-1735 UV induced melanoma and its metastases, *Cancer Immunol. Immunother.*, 15, 11, 1983.

158. Foley, E. J., Antigen properties of methylcholanthrene-induced tumors in mice of strain of origin, *Cancer Res.*, 13, 835, 1953.

159. Rubinstein, P., Decary, F., and Streun, E. W., Quantitative studies on tumor enhancement in mice. I. Enhancement of sarcoma 1 induced by IgM, IgG, and IgG$_2$, *J. Exp. Med.*, 140, 591, 1974.

160. Klein, G. and Klein, E., Rejectability of virus-induced tumors and nonrejectability of spontaneous tumors: a lesson in contrasts, *Transplant. Proc.*, 9, 1095, 1977.

161. Weiss, D. W., The questionable immunogenicity of certain neoplasms. What then the prospects for immunological intervention in malignant disease?, *Cancer Immunol. Immunother.*, 2, 11, 1977.

162. Haagensen, D. E., Roloson, G., Collins, J. J., Wells, S. A., Bolognesi, D. P., and Harsen, H. J., Immunologic control of the ascites form of murine adenocarcinoma 755. I. Protection with syngeneic immune serum of lymphoid cells, *J. Natl. Cancer Inst.*, 60, 131, 1978.

163. Pollack, S., Specific 'arming' of normal lymph node cells by sera from tumour-bearing mice, *Int. J. Cancer*, 11, 138, 1973.

164. Kohler, G. and Milstein, C., Continuous cultures of fused cells secreting antibody of pre-defined specificity, *Nature (London)*, 256, 495, 1975.

165. Larson, S. M., Brown, J. P., Wright, P. W., Carrasquillo, J. A., Hellstrom, I., and Hellstrom, K. W., Imaging of melanoma with ^{131}I-labeled monoclonal antibodies, *J. Nucl. Med.*, 24, 123, 1983.

166. Gatter, K. C., Abdulaziz, Z., Beverley, P., Corvalan, J. R. F., Ford, C., Lane, E. G., Mota, M., Nash, J. R. G., Pulford, K., Stein, H., Taylor-Papadimitriou, J., Woodhouse, C., and Mason, D. Y., Use of monoclonal antibodies for the histopathobiological diagnosis of human malignancy, *J. Clin. Pathol.*, 35, 1253, 1982.

167. McGee, J. O'D., Woods, J. C., Ashall, F., Bramwell, M. E., and Harris, H., A new marker for human cancer cells. II. Immunohistochemical detection of the Ca antigen in human tissue with the Ca₁ antibody, *Lancet,* ii, 7, 1982.

168. Brown, J. P., Woodbury, R. G., Hart, C. E., Hellstrom, K. E., Quantitative analysis of melanoma-associated antigen p97 in normal and neoplastic tissues, *Proc. Natl. Acad. Sci. U.S.A.,* 78, 539, 1981.

169. Menard, S., Tagliabue, E., Canevari, S., Fossati, G., and Calnaghi, M. I., Generation of monoclonal antibodies reacting with normal and cancer cells of human breast, *Cancer Res.,* 43, 1295, 1983.

170. Ceriani, R. P., Peterson, J. A., and Blank, E. W., Variability in surface antigen expression of human breast epithelial cells cultured from normal breast, normal tissue peripheral to breast carcinomas, and breast carcinomas, *Cancer Res.,* 44, 3033, 1984.

171. Edwards, P. A. W., Heterogeneous expression of cell-surface antigens in normal epithelia and their tumours, revealed by monoclonal antibodies, *Br. J. Cancer,* 51, 149, 1985.

172. Bramwell, M. E., Bhavanandan, V. P., Wiseman, G., and Harris, H., Structure and function of the Ca antigen, *Br. J. Cancer,* 48, 177, 1983.

173. Burchell, J., Durbin, H., and Taylor-Papadimitriou, J., Complexity of expression of antigenic determinants, recognized by monoclonal antibodies HMFG1 and HMFG-2, in normal and malignant human mammary epithelial cells, *J. Immunol.,* 131, 508, 1983.

174. Magnani, J. L., Brockhaus, M., Smith, D. F., Ginsburg, V., Blaszyk, M., Mitchell, K. F., Steplewski, Z., and Koprowski, H., A monosialoganglioside is a monoclonal antibody-defined antigen of colon carcinoma, *Science,* 212, 55, 1981.

175. Rettig, W. J., Cordon-Cardo, C., Ng, J. S. C., Oettgen, H. F., Old, L. J., and Lloyd, K. O., High molecular weight glycoproteins of human teratocarcinoma defined by monoclonal antibodies to carbohydrate determinants, *Cancer Res.,* 45, 815, 1985.

176. Bremer, E. G., Levery, S. B., Sonnino, S., Ghidani, R., Canevari, S., Konnagi, R., and Hakomori, S. I., Characterization of a glycosphingolipid antigen defined by the monoclonal antibody MBr1 expressed in normal and neoplastic epithelial cells of human mammary gland, *J. Biol. Chem.,* 259, 14773, 1984.

177. Bernstein, I. D., Tay, M. R., and Nowinski, R. C., Mouse leukemia: therapy with monoclonal antibodies inhibit tumor growth against a thymus differentiation antigen, *Science,* 207, 87, 1979.

178. Kirch, M. E. and Hammerling, V., Immunotherapy of murine leukemias by monoclonal antibody. I. Effect of passively administered antibody on growth of transplanted tumor cells, *J. Immunol.,* 127, 805, 1981.

179. Nadler, L. M., Stashenko, P., Hardy, R., Kaplan, W. D., Buttan, L. N., Kufe, D. W., Antman, K. H., and Schlossman, S. F., Serotherapy of a patient with a monoclonal antibody directed against a human lymphoma-associated antigen, *Cancer Res.,* 40, 3147, 1980.

180. Miller, R. A., Maloney, D. E., McKillop, J., and Levy, R., *In vivo* effects of murine hybridoma monoclonal antibody in a patient with T-cell leukemia, *Blood,* 58, 78, 1981.

181. Ritz, J., Pesandro, J. M., Sallen, S. E., Clavell, L. A., Notis-McConarty, J., Rosenthal, P., and Schlossman, S. F., Serotherapy of acute lymphoblastic leukemia with monoclonal antibody, *Blood,* 58, 141, 1981.

182. Miller, R. A., Maloney, D. E., Warnke, R., and Levy, R., Treatment of B cell lymphoma with monoclonal anti-idiotype antibody, *N. Engl. J. Med.,* 306, 517, 1982.

183. North, S. M. and Dean, C. J., Monoclonal antibodies to rat sarcomata. II. A syngeneic IgG₂ᵦ antibody with anti-tumor activity, *Immunology,* 49, 667, 1983.

184. North, S. M., Styles, J. M., Hobbs, S. M., and Dean, C. J., Monoclonal antibodies to rat sarcomata. I. Mode of immunization and tumour specificity, *Immunology,* 47, 397, 1982.

185. Herlyn, D. and Koprowski, H., IgG₂ₐ monoclonal antibodies inhibit tumor growth through interaction with effector cells, *Proc. Natl. Acad. Sci. U.S.A.,* 79, 4761, 1982.

186. Jerne, N. K., Towards a network theory of the immune system, *Ann. Immunol. (Institute Pasteur),* 125C, 373, 1974.

187. Jerry, L. M., Rowden, G., Cano, P. O., Phillips, T. M., Deutsch, G. F., Capek, A., Hartman, D., and Lewis, M. G., Immune complexes in human melanoma: a consequence of deranged immune regulation, *Scand. J. Immunol.,* 5, 845, 1976.

188. Winchester, R. J., Kunkel, H. G., and Agnello, V., Occurrence of globulin complexes in serum and joint fluid of rheumatoid arthritis patients: use of monoclonal rheumatoid factors as reagents for their demonstration, *J. Exp. Med.,* 134, 2286, 1972.

189. Beatty, P. G., Kim, B. S., Rowley, D. A., and Coppleson, L. W., Antibody against the antigen receptor of a plasmacytoma prolongs survival of mice bearing the tumor, *J. Immunol.,* 116, 1391, 1976.

190. Lewis, M. G., Hartman, D., and Jerry, L. M., Antibodies and anti-antibodies in human malignancy: an expression of deranged immune regulation, *Ann. N.Y. Acad. Sci.,* 276, 316, 1976.

191. Schlom, J., Wunderlich, D., and Teramoto, Y. A., Generation of human monoclonal antibodies reactive with human mammary carcinoma cells, *Proc. Natl. Acad. Sci. U.S.A.,* 77, 23, 1980.

192. Koprowski, H., Herlyn, D., Lubeck, M., Defreitos, E., and Steplewski, H. F., Human anti-idiotype antibodies in cancer patients: is the modulation of the immune response beneficial for the patients?, *Proc. Natl. Acad. Sci. U.S.A.,* 81, 216, 1984.

193. Brunhouse, R. and Cebra, J. J., Isotypes of IgG: comparison of the primary structures of three pairs of isotypes which differ in their ability to activate complement, *Mol. Immunol.,* 16, 907, 1979.

194. Der Balian, G. P., Slack, J., Clevinger, B. L., Bazin, H., and Davie, J. M., Subclass restriction of murine antibodies. III. Antigens that stimulate IgG_3 in mice stimulate IgG_{2c} in rats, *J. Exp. Med.,* 152, 209, 1980.

195. Mosier, J. E., Ming, J. J., and Goldings, E. A., The ontogeny of thymic independent antibody response *in vitro* in normal mice and mice with an X-linked B cell defect, *J. Immunol.,* 119, 1874, 1977.

196. McKearn, J. P. and Quintians, J., Ontogeny of murine B cell responses to thymus-independent trinitophenyl antigens, *Cell. Immunol.,* 44, 367, 1979.

197. Nahm, M., Der-Balian, G. P., Venturini, D., Bazin, H., and Davie, J. M., Antigenic similarities of rat and mouse IgG subclass associated with anti-carbohydrate specificities, *Immunogenetics,* 11, 199, 1980.

198. Perlmutter, R. M., Hansburg, D., Briles, D. E., Nicolotti, R. A., and Davie, J. M., Subclass restriction of murine anti-carbohydrate antibodies, *J. Immunol.,* 121, 566, 1978.

199. Lewis, G. K. and Goodman, J. W., Carrier-directed anti-hapten responses by B-cell subsets, *J. Exp. Med.,* 146, 1, 1977.

200. Unkeless, J. C., The presence of two Fc receptors on mouse macrophages: evidence from a variant cell line and differential trypsin sensitivity, *J. Exp. Med.,* 145, 931, 1977.

201. Diamond, B. and Yelton, D. E., A new Fc receptor on mouse macrophage binding IgG_3, *J. Exp. Med.,* 153, 514, 1981.

Chapter 2

ANTIGENIC HETEROGENEITY IN METASTASIS

Fred R. Miller and Gloria H. Heppner

TABLE OF CONTENTS

I. INTRODUCTION

Although host immunity can influence the metastatic spread of tumor cells, the extent, and even the direction, of that influence varies with different tumors. Fidler et al.[1] found that a strongly antigenic tumor was more metastatic in immunosuppressed than in normal mice, whereas a weakly immunogenic tumor was less metastatic in the immunocompromised hosts. Any discussion of the role of immunity in malignancy must be tempered with the realization that the multiple parameters involved in both phenomena preclude definitive generalizations. Every tumor, and every tumor-host relationship, is but a single example of an extremely complex set of interacting and interwoven factors. The concepts of tumor heterogeneity can help provide a framework for these complexities. The purpose of this paper is to illustrate the range of possible relationships between immunity and metastasis, not to review all the many examples that can be found in the literature.

A growing appreciation of the cellular heterogeneity within tumors has led to a large number of studies in which characteristics of tumor subpopulations that metastasize at a high frequency have been compared with those of poorly metastatic subpopulations. These attempts to identify the unique characteristics of the metastatic phenotype have frequently focused on cell surface properties of the tumor cells. The concept of immune surveillance is often extended to suggest that metastatic subpopulations are more resistant to host defense mechanisms than are nonmetastatic, albeit progressively growing, cells in the primary tumor. The repeated observations of antigenic and immunogenic heterogeneity within primary tumors is consonant with the hypothesis that metastasis results from a tumor cell subfraction which is able to escape the defense reactions of the host.[2,3]

The notion of a "metastatic cascade", in which tumor cells must be able to complete multiple steps in order to form metastases,[4,5] is widely accepted and now seems obvious. The immunological consequences of the cascade are less obvious: investigators will describe the steps which must be accomplished by the metastatic cell and then express amazement that a nonmetastatic tumor line appears to be immunologically inert. Even if the concept of immune surveillance is applicable to the process of metastasis, immunological escape would be only one of the multiple number of steps that need be achieved; cells which had failed to make some of the necessary "adaptations" (whether genetic or epigenetic) to be metastatic might still have become neutral immunologically. Thus, "nonmetastatic" subpopulations may be incapable of provoking an effective immune response; indeed, the metastatic cascade concept predicts this will be the case at least some of the time. As the following review will show, however, this view is also much too simple to explain the range of immunological relationships that have been observed between primary and metastatic tumors and between high and low metastatic subpopulations.

II. IMMUNOLOGIC DISPARITY BETWEEN PRIMARY TUMORS AND METASTASES

Rodent sarcomas induced by treatment with methylcholanthrene (MCA) have been used by several investigators to study immunologic heterogeneity between primary tumors and their metastases. Kodama et al.[6] selected two metastatic variants, one from a lymph node metastasis and one from the lung. As assessed by the effects of X-ray induced immunosuppression and OK 432 immunostimulation, the parental mouse sarcoma was more immunogenic than either metastatic line. However, such results are not typical. Sugarbaker and Cohen selected 7 of 18 lung metastases (M2, M6, M9, M10, M13, M15, M16) which had growth rates similar to that of the primary (P).[7] Two of the metastatic lines were neither immunogenic nor antigenic; neither M10 nor M15 could immunize against either themselves or against P, and P did not immunize against them. On the other hand, two other metastatic lines were not demonstrably different from P; both M13 and M16 immunized against themselves and against P, and P immunized against both M13 and M16. The other three metastatic lines had unique immunologic characteristics. M2 immunized against itself and P, but P did not immunize against M2 challenge. M6 was antigenic but not immunogenic; animals immunized to P, but not to M6, were resistant to M6. M9 immunized against itself, but cross-reactivity with P was not seen. Thus, every imaginable combination of immunogenic characteristics between the primary and a metastasis was demonstrated in this one sarcoma. Faraci found that a parental MCA-induced mouse fibrosarcoma and two lung metastases were all able to immunize against themselves and against the other two lines.[8] With an MCA-induced rat fibrosarcoma, Pimm et al.[9] also demonstrated that metastases were immunologically indistinguishable from the primary. A subline from a lung metastasis and a subline from a kidney metastasis were not cross reactive with the primary or peritoneal metastasis but were reciprocally cross-reactive with each other. Wang et al.[10] compared the immunogenicity, antigenicity, and metastatic ability of a parental MCA induced mouse sarcoma and three clones (clone 10, clone 27, and clone 34). The most metastatic clone (clone 10) and the parental tumor were equally immunogenic; the other two clones were weaker immunogens. Clone 34 was intermediate between the parental tumor and clone 10 in its ability to metastasize and clone 27 was less metastatic. From the pattern of cross-protection between the lines in the study, Wang et al.[10] proposed a model involving four determinants expressed differentially on the three clones. One antigen was shared by clones 10 and 27, one shared by clones 10 and 34, one unique to clone 27, and one unique to clone 34. Thus, although some common antigens were expressed by multiple populations, no antigen was shared by all the cells.

Proctor et al.[11] found that a rat benzo(α)pyrene(BP)-induced sarcoma, a lymph node metastasis, and two lung metastases were equally able to immunize rats against subsequent i.v. challenge with any of the four lines. Sugarbaker et al.[12] also studied a rat BP-induced fibrosarcoma. They compared the parental (P) and two lung metastases (M0 and M1). P, M0, and M1 immunized animals to subsequent challenge with the tumor used for immunization. M0 and M1 immunized animals to P and weakly to each other (latency increased but no change in final incidence). P did not immunize rats against either M0 or M1. Thus, the lines established from lung metastases seemed somewhat less antigenic than the parental line. However, the parental tumor was as metastatic as M0 and M1. Similarly, Mantovani et al.[13] compared cell lines from nine individual lung metastases of a BP-induced mouse sarcoma. Some were more metastatic than the parental line, some were less metastatic, and some the same. Mice immunized with the parental tumor were resistant to challenge with seven of the nine lines established from metastases. The two lines which were not antigenic (i.e., preimmunization with parental cells did not affect their growth) were not immunogenic either — they did not immunize against themselves. Of these two lines, one was less metastatic than the parental cells and one was the same.

Several cell lines and clones from primary Lewis lung carcinoma (3LL) implants growing subcutaneously and from their lung metastases were found by Kiger to differ in expression of H-2 antigens and of a tumor associated antigen (TAA) detectable with a monoclonal antibody.[14] The expression of these antigens did not correlate with frequency of metastasis. Previous work with a 3LL line established from a local subcutaneous tumor (L-3LL) and a line established from a lung metastasis (M-3LL) indicated that each induced specific immunity and was not cross-reactive.[15] Brodt and Segal prepared 3M KCl extracts of L-3LL and M-3LL and used the extracts to "educate'' macrophages in vitro.[16] These macrophages were adoptively transferred to mice. Macrophages treated with extracts of L-3LL protected mice from the growth of L-3LL (but not of M-3LL) in the subcutis and inhibited metastasis from the primary. Macrophages treated with extracts of M-3LL had no effect on the growth or metastasis of either M-3LL or L-3LL. However, M-3LL tumors were not more metastatic than L-3LL tumors.

By using panels of monoclonal antibodies, antigenic heterogeneity between primary tumors and metastases has been seen in man. Primus et al.[17] used four monoclonal antibodies to carcinoembryonic antigen (CEA) in a study of human colonic carcinoma patients. One of those, monoclonal NP-4, rarely stained nodal or liver metastases even though up to 90% of the cells in the primary were positive. In a study of 81 gastric cancer patients with metastatic deposits in lymph nodes, Hockey et al.[18] found that metastases from CEA negative primaries could be CEA positive and that metastases from CEA positive primaries were sometimes CEA negative. In 12 of 60 patients with more than 1 metastasis, the metastases were heterogeneous, with at least 1 CEA positive and 1 CEA negative node. Roth et al.[19] studied 15 human sarcomas with a panel of 4 monoclonal antibodies. Primary tumors and metastatic nodules were often dissimilar. A metastasis could be positive while the primary was negative and vice versa. Not all metastases from a single patient reacted uniformly with the panel of monoclonals. In an earlier study, Roth and Wesley demonstrated that butanol extracted antigen from both primaries and metastases reacted with the patients' serum.[20] Primary cells were better able to inhibit this reaction competitively than were cells from metastases.

III. DISPARITY BETWEEN RESISTANCE TO PRIMARY GROWTH AND TO METASTASES FROM THE PRIMARY TUMOR

Pot-Deprun et al.[21] induced a rhabdomyosarcoma in a rat by implanting nickel intramuscularly. The primary tumor was cultured in vitro and several clones were derived. The parental, uncloned tumor was both immunogenic and antigenic. Preimmunization with irradiated cells resulted in diminished incidence of tumors and increased survival of the rats which did develop tumors after the challenge transplant. However, preimmunization did not protect the rats from metastasis from tumors growing subcutaneously. In fact, preimmunized rats which developed tumors had significantly more metastases in the lung than did the control rats. Of eight clones tested, all of which were metastatic, two immunized rats by the subcutaneous challenge transplantation assay but only one also protected against metastases. Pretreatment with a third clone caused enhanced growth of the subcutaneous challenge transplant and increased metastasis: five clones were not immunogenic. These authors felt that, because "immunization did not protect rats from pulmonary metastasis, . . . the metastasizing cells may originate in a nonimmunogenic cell population". Cells from the metastases occurring in preimmunized rats were not, however, tested for immunologic properties.

Conversely, Yu et al.[22] found that clones of an MCA-induced mouse sarcoma could immunize mice more effectively against metastasis than against growth in the subcutis. Mice were preimmunized with the parental tumor or one of three clones, and then challenged with a large number of cells so that both immunized and control mice would develop comparable s.c. tumors. The preimmunized mice had significantly fewer metastases than the control mice. The specificity of cross-protection to metastasis was identical to that which could be demonstrated with lower numbers of challenge tumor cells injected subcutaneously.[10]

IV. IMMUNOLOGIC HETEROGENEITY OF TUMOR SUBPOPULATIONS SELECTED FOR HIGH AND LOW FREQUENCY OF METASTASIS

As previously discussed, lines established from a primary tumor and from metastases of that tumor are often both metastatic. Thus, differences in immunologic properties between the two might be expected to be minimal. A common procedure to maximize differences has been to select low- and high-metastatic variants.

The F1 and F10 variants of the mouse B16 melanoma are of low- and high-metastatic phenotypes, respectively. The F10 subpopulation has been shown to induce a higher antibody titer than F1.[23] Tumors were removed from syngeneic mice and treated with 0.12 *M* citrate buffer at pH 3.5 to elute immunoglobulin bound to the cell surface. More immunoglobulin could be eluted from F10 tumor cells than from F1 tumor cells. It was not shown that the eluted immunoglobulin was tumor specific, however. Crude butanol extracts of F1 and F10 were prepared by Legrue and Hearn.[24] Immunization with the F1 preparation protected mice from both F1 and F10 challenge whether the challenge cells were injected s.c. or i.v. The F10 preparation did not induce resistance to s.c. challenge with either F1 or F10 cells. In fact, pretreatment with F10 extract enhanced lung colonization by F10 cells after i.v. injection.

Our own studies with subpopulations of a single, spontaneously arising BALB/cfC$_3$H mouse mammary tumor indicate that immunologic and metastatic characteristics are not necessarily linked. Subpopulations 66 and 410.4 are highly metastatic. Subpopulation 66 is neither immunogenic nor antigenic whereas preimmunization with 410.4 induces resistance to both s.c. and i.v. challenge.[25] A third subpopulation, 168, does not metastasize spontaneously from the subcutis but is nearly as efficient as 66 and 410.4 in lung colonization after i.v. injection.[26] Subpopulation 168 is not immunogenic but is detectably antigenic, being unable to immunize mice to itself, but preimmunization with the nonmetastatic subpopulation 410 renders mice resistant to challenge with 168 cells.[27] These tumor subpopulations also induce characteristic lymphocytic infiltrates in vivo,[28] but no correlation between these infiltrates and the metastatic phenotype is seen. On the other hand, those tumors that are able to metastasize spontaneously are infiltrated with a higher proportion of mature, activated macrophages than are nonmetastatic tumors.[29] Line 168 tumors are intermediate in levels of activated, infiltrating macrophages.[30]

A nonmetastatic variant (Eb) and a metastatic variant (ESb) of the L5178Y lymphoma are equally able to induce a T-cell lytic response and to be lysed by cytotoxic T-cells in a chromium-release test.[31] Eb and ESb are not cross-reactive. In experiments in which the cytotoxic T-cells were prepared by sensitization in vivo and secondary stimulation of splenocytes in vitro with mitomycin-C treated tumor cells, it was necessary for the tumor cells used both for in vivo sensitization and in vitro stimulation to be homologous with the target cells. When evaluated by resistance to transplantation challenge, TAA of Eb and ESb were again found to be specific. However, immunity to Eb induced by Eb was stronger than the immunity induced to ESb by ESb.[32] Fogel et al.[33] selected an ESb variant which was adherent to plastic (ESb-M) and was not metastatic. As judged by the chromium-release assay, ESb and ESb-M expressed the same TAA and the same differentiation antigens. The two variants did, however, bind different lectins and revertant, metastatic ESb-M cells bound the same lectins as ESb. After neuraminidase treatment, ESb bound the same lectins as ESb-M. Thus, the differences between ESb and ESb-M were due to sialic acid "masking" of the lectin binding sites. Altevogt et al.[34] found that the metastatic and nonmetastatic variants had similar amounts of sialic acid and the same lectin binding sites, but the sialic acid masked different lectin binding sites in the variant lines. Simmons and Rios have similarly reported that neuraminidase treatment differentially enhances expression of some tumor antigens (tumor specific transplantation antigens) but not others (MTV-viral antigens).[35] Altevogt et al.[34] also studied high- and low-metastic variants of the MDAY-D2 lymphoma and found that the low-metastatic line had less total sialic acid.

Tao and Burger selected B16 melanoma variants for resistance to ricin and wheat germ agglutinin.[36] Selected variants were rarely metastatic from intramuscular primaries and were inefficient in forming lung colonies after i.v. injection. Selection for Con A resistance did not concomitantly select for a low metastatic phenotype but, rather, for a variant with increased incidence of metastatic nodules in the liver after i.v. injection. On the other hand, Reading et al.[37] did not find a correlation between Con A binding or WGA binding and metastasis of RAW 117 variants. They did, however, describe an inverse relationship between experimental liver metastasis and expression of Moloney MLV gp70. In other cases Con A binding has correlated with metastasis. Cells from pulmonary nodules bound less Con A than cells from parental, spontaneous mouse mammary tumors.[38] Hagmar and Ryd described two forms of a mouse squamous cell carcinoma;[39] one that metastasized to the lung and one that metastasized to extra-pulmonary sites. By enzymatic dispersion, the form metastasizing to the lung became metastatic to extrapulmonary sites instead. The two original forms were distinctly different in their abilities to agglutinate with Con A and WGA, a distinction which was retained after enzymatic treatment. Thus, differences in these two lectin binding sites were not correlated with organ selectivity of metastases.

Shearman and Longenecker reported the presence of a liver metastasis-associated antigen (LMAA) on subpopulations of a chicken T-cell lymphoma induced by Marek's disease virus.[40] AL2 was a selected liver metastasis variant and AL3 was selected for ovarian metastases. Both lines were then used to derive several clones which metastasized to the liver (of chick embryos) at various frequencies. Binding of a monoclonal antibody to LMAA correlated with the number of liver metastases. Shearman et al.[41] demonstrated that anti-LMAA monoclonal antibody inhibited liver metastasis formation in this system.

V. EFFECTS OF IMMUNOSELECTION ON METASTATIC PHENOTYPE

The above section describes studies in which investigators compared the immunological properties of cells selected for high- vs. low-metastatic frequency. A related "mirror-image" approach is to compare the metastatic properties of cells selected for differences in immunological parameters. Fidler and associates cocultured the B16 melanoma lines F1 and F10 in vitro for 7 to 10 days with lymphocytes from mice immunized against B16.[42] This procedure was repeated six times for each line and the resultant selected variants were designated F1-Lr6 and F10-Lr6. Subcutaneous growth of the lymphocyte resistant variants did not differ from that of the unselected lines. However, after i.v. injection the lymphocyte resistant variants were less efficient at forming lung colonies than were their respective, unselected lines.

Coculture of ESb cells with anti-ESb cytotoxic T-lymphocytes (CTLs) did not select for immunoresistant ESb cells.[43] However, cells from metastases which developed from ESb tumors growing subcutaneously gradually lost sensitivity to anti-ESb CTLs.[43] The loss occurred faster in the spleen than in the lung, brain, and liver metastases.[44] Sensitivity to anti-Eb CTLs was not acquired and sensitivity to ant-H2^d or anti-H2^K CTLs was not changed. Bosslet and Schirrmacher found that the cells from splenic metastases nodules (ESb$_{MET-SPL}$) were not active in cold inhibition assays and neuraminidase treatment did not alter the lack of TATA expression.[44] The characteristic was stable through 100 cell generations in tissue culture. The ESB$_{MET-SPL}$ did not generate CTLs. If ESb cells were injected s.c. into nude mice, the cells from splenic metastases were still immunogenic. The fact that cells from metastatic nodules were initially sensitive to anti-ESb CTLs indicates that the selection process occurred after metastasis rather than as a prerequisite.

A metastatic clone of sarcoma T10, which was induced with MCA in an F1 $H2^b \times H2^K$ mouse, was immunoselected in vivo by growth in semi-allogeneic mice.[45] The original clone expressed both $H2^b$ and $H2^K$. Variants that had lost both $H2^b$ and $H2^K$ were no longer metastatic. Those variants with only $H2^b$ loss were more metastatic than the unselected parental clone. The H2 phenotypes of the selected cells were stable when transplanted back into syngeneic F1 mice. In an earlier report, DeBaitselier et al.[46] isolated ten clones of the T10 sarcoma. All clones expressed $H2^b$ but only two strongly expressed $H2^K$. Those two clones were efficient in lung colonization. Thus, $H2^K$ directly correlated with metastasis in this system.

By contrast, studies of clones of the Lewis lung carcinoma line indicated that $H2^K$ is inversely correlated with metastasis.[47,48] In a study of 30 Lewis lung carcinoma clones, a low $H2^K/H2^d$ ratio correlated with high metastatic phenotype.[47] A highly metastatic clone (D122) and a poorly metastatic clone (A9) were studied further.[48] The poorly metastatic A9 expressed $H2^K$ as well as $H2^D$ and was both immunogenic and antigenic. The highly metastic D122 expressed only $H2^D$ and was antigenic (preimmunization with A9 protected mice from challenge with D122) but was not immunogenic. Eisenbach et al.[48] proposed that the display of TAA with $H2^D$ induces suppressor cells and that the display of TAA with $H2^K$ induces immunity.

VI. ANTIGENIC HETEROGENEITY IN METASTASIS — SO WHAT?

It is clear from a large number of studies that both animal and human cancers are antigenically and immunogenically heterogeneous. Such heterogeneity can be seen within primary tumors, within metastases, and between primary tumors and their metastases. The question to be addressed is whether this immunological heterogeneity is causally related to the development of metastasis or whether immunological heterogeneity and metastases are independent manifestations of the same loss of control mechanisms that otherwise regulate genetic and phenotypic diversification. Our review of the literature suggests that there are no general rules that apply to the immune response and the process of metastasis. Examples of every sort of relationship between antigenicity/immunogenicity and metastasis can be cited, often times within the same tumor. Before accepting that the immune response is irrelevant to metastasis, however, one must consider the limitations of the methods used to demonstrate both immunologic and metastatic heterogeneity within tumor populations.

If one takes a tumor and disassembles it into component subpopulations, those subpopulations will differ in many properties. Both immunologic properties and metastatic properties can be determined for the subpopulations, but the ability of the intact, autochthonous tumor to induce a host response is not thereby reproduced. The establishment of a metastatic nodule in an autochthonous host occurs after a cancer progresses through several cellular generations with, presumably, a continuous generation of new variant subpopulations. Each new subpopulation may stimulate the immune system, but the immunological status of the host is already a complex result of all previous stimuli. The immunologic and metastatic characteristics of an isolated subpopulation (if its source is an inbred experimental animal) are easily determined in normal syngeneic or in preimmunized animals but it is impossible to reproduce the immune state of the original host at the time that subpopulation evolved and metastasized. Even simple experiments, in which the interactions between pairs of subpopulations have been studied in previously nonstimulated hosts, indicate that interactions can occur which mask both the immunologic and metastatic phenotypes of individual subpopulations.

Mixtures of two sublines of the TA3 mouse mammary adenocarcinoma, injected into normal mice at various ratios, resulted in either the growth of both lines or the rejection of both lines depending upon which subline was in excess.[49] Descriptions of "one-way cross reactivity" between tumor subpopulations suggest that the inability of a subpopulation to induce immunity may be irrelevant in the autochthonous host if that subpopulation is sensitive to a host response induced by a sister subpopulation.[7,27,50-52] Alternatively, an antigen hierarchy may exist such that a response to one antigen precludes a response to a second antigen. Urban et al.[53] found that an otherwise immunogenic antigen may not induce an immune response in the presence of a response to an "immuno dominant" antigen. The UV-irradiation-induced fibrosarcoma 1591 usually regresses (1591-RE) in normal syngeneic mice but in rare instances it grows progressively (1591-PRO). Immunization with 1591-RE induces CTLs only against 1591-RE. Immunization with 1591-PRO induces CTLs against both 1591-RE and 1591-PRO. Thus, 1591-RE has two TAAs but only one is immunogenic. 1591-PRO has lost the TAA which is immunogenic on 1591-RE but the second TAA, non-immunogenic but antigenic in 1591-RE, is immunogenic as expressed in 1591-PRO.

Not only are immunological properties subject to modifications by subpopulation interactions, metastatic phenotypes of isolated subpopulations are also influenced by co-existence with other subpopulations. Miller has reported that the simultaneous presence of metastatic and nonmetastatic subpopulations of a mouse mammary tumor can result in metastatic nodules containing clonogenic cells of the nonmetastatic subpopulation.[54,55] Thus, the methods used to demonstrate cellular heterogeneity within tumors can only show that heterogeneity exists. They cannot predict the impact of that heterogeneity on the behavior of "whole" tumors.

Tumor heterogeneity is the result of a dynamic process by which new variants are generated from unstable stem cells. The process does not end when metastasis occurs or when a cell line is established in tissue culture or as a transplantable line. Thus, what is isolated from a metastatic nodule may not closely resemble the cell(s) which originally metastasized from a primary tumor. Furthermore, both antigen expression and metastatic characteristics can be cell cycle dependent,[56-59] but antigen expression can also fluctuate independently of the cell cycle in a nonheritable manner.[60,61] Antigen expression can also be altered by therapeutic intervention with chemotherapeutic agents or with biological response modifiers.[62,63] The generation of metastatic heterogeneity is influenced by interactions between existing tumor subpopulations,[64] and the stability of the metastatic phenotype is itself heterogeneous for different tumors,[10,65,66] as well as for different subpopulations of the same tumor.[26]

Regardless of the biological significance of the antigenic heterogeneity of tumors, it is likely to have considerable practical consequences. In so far as antigens and immunogens are distributed heterogeneously among tumor populations they pose a problem for immunodetection and immunotherapy. The response of metastatic disease to a given immunological intervention cannot be predicted on the basis of knowledge about the immunologic properties of the primary tumor. The very feature which makes immunological approaches to cancer control so appealing, namely the specificity of immune reactivity, makes it especially vulnerable to the problems of tumor heterogeneity. Here, as for related problems in chemotherapy,[67] it is necessary to consider combinations of therapies, designed for multiple targets. Immunological heterogeneity may, or may not, play a biological role in metastasis, but its role in circumventing detection and treatment certainly contributes to the clinical progression of neoplastic disease.

ACKNOWLEDGMENTS

The authors wish to thank Margaret Peterson for typing this manuscript and to acknowledge the support of the Concern Foundation.

REFERENCES

1. Fidler, I. J., Gersten, D. M., and Kripke, M. L., Influence of immune status on the metastasis of three murine fibrosarcomas of different immunogenicities, *Cancer Res.*, 39, 3816, 1979.
2. Kerbel, R. S., Implications of immunological heterogeneity of tumours, *Nature (London)*, 280, 358, 1979.
3. Miller, F. R., Intratumor immunologic heterogeneity, *Cancer Met. Rev.*, 1, 319, 1982.
4. Fidler, I. J., Tumor heterogeneity and the biology of cancer invasion and metastasis, *Cancer Res.*, 38, 2651, 1978.
5. Poste, G. and Fidler, I. J., The pathogenesis of cancer metastasis, *Nature (London)*, 283, 139, 1980.
6. Kodama, Y., Seyama, T., Kamiya, K., and Yokoro, K., Establishment and immunological characterization of 3-methylcholanthrene-induced sarcoma cell lines metastasizing widely in mice and exhibiting distinct and selective propensities for the mode of metastasis, *J. Natl. Cancer Inst.*, 69, 595, 1982.
7. Sugarbaker, E. V. and Cohen, A. M., Altered antigenicity in spontaneous pulmonary metastases from an antigenic murine sarcoma, *Surgery*, 72, 155, 1972.
8. Faraci, R. P., In vitro demonstration of altered antigenicity of metastases from a primary methylcholanthrene-induced sarcoma, *Surgery*, 76, 469, 1974.
9. Pimm, M. V., Embleton, M. J., and Baldwin, R. W., Multiple antigenic specificities within primary 3-methylcholanthrene-induced rat sarcomas and metastases, *Int. J. Cancer*, 25, 621, 1980.
10. Wang, N., Yu, S. H., Liener, I. E., Hebbel, R. P., Eaton, J. W., and McKhann, C. F., Characterization of high- and low-metastatic clones derived from a methylcholanthrene-induced murine fibrosarcoma, *Cancer Res.*, 42, 1046, 1982.
11. Proctor, J. W., Palmer, P., and Rudenstam, C.-M., Transplantation isoantigenicity of a rat sarcoma and its spontaneous metastases, *J. Natl. Cancer Inst.*, 53, 579, 1974.
12. Sugarbaker, E. V., Cohen, A. M., and Ketcham, A. S., Concomitant tumor immunity and immunoselection of metastases, *Curr. Top. Surg.*, 3, 349, 1971.
13. Mantovani, A., Giavazzi, R., Alessandri, G., Spreafico, F., and Garattini, S., Characterization of tumor lines derived from spontaneous metastases of a transplanted murine sarcoma, *Eur. J. Cancer*, 17, 71, 1981.
14. Kiger, N., Heterogeneity in surface antigen of cell lines and clones from a murine carcinoma, *Int. J. Cancer*, 35, 129, 1985.
15. Fogel, M., Gorelik, E., Segal, S., and Feldman, M., Differences in cell surface antigens of tumor metastases and those of the local tumor, *J. Natl. Cancer Inst.*, 62, 585, 1979.
16. Brodt, P. and Segal, S., Differences in immunogenicity between the local tumor 3LL and its metastasis-derived line as detected by sensitization with antigen-fed macrophages, *Invasion Met.*, 2, 185, 1982.
17. Primus, F. J., Kuhns, W. J., and Goldenberg, D. M., Immunological heterogeneity of carcinoembryonic antigen: immunohistochemical detection of carcinoembryonic antigen determinants in colonic tumors with monoclonal antibodies, *Cancer Res.*, 43, 693, 1983.
18. Hockey, M. C., Stokes, H. J., Thompson, H., Woodhouse, C. S., Macdonald, F., Fielding, J. W. L., and Ford, C. H. J., Carcinoembryonic antigen (CEA) expression and heterogeneity in primary and autologous metastatic gastric tumours demonstrated by a monoclonal antibody, *Br. J. Cancer*, 49, 129, 1984.
19. Roth, J. A., Restrepo, C., Scuderi, P., Baldwin, R. W., Reichert. C. M., and Hosoi, S., Analysis of antigenic expression by primary and autologous metastatic human sarcomas using murine monoclonal antibodies, *Cancer Res.*, 44, 5320, 1984.
20. Roth, J. A. and Wesley, R. A., Human tumor-associated antigens detected by serological techniques: analysis of autologous humoral immune responses to primary and metastatic human sarcomas by an enzyme-linked immunoabsorbant solid-phase assay (ELISA), *Cancer Res.*, 42, 3978, 1982.
21. Pot-Deprun, J., Poupon, M. F., Sweeney, F. L., and Chouroulinteov, I., Growth, metastasis, immunogenicity, and chromosomal content of a nickel-induced rhabdomyosarcoma and subsequent cloned cell lines in rats, *J. Natl. Cancer Inst.*, 71, 1241, 1983.
22. Yu, S., Wang, N., and McKhann, C. F., The effect of immunity on pulmonary metastasis of a methylcholanthrene-induced fibrosarcoma and three of its clones, *J. Surg. Oncol.*, 27, 51, 1984.
23. Baniyash, M., Smorodinsky, N. I., Yaakubovicz, M., and Witz, I. P., Serologically detectable MHC and tumor-associated antigens on B16 melanoma variants and humoral immunity in mice bearing these tumors, *J. Immunol.*, 129, 1318, 1982.
24. LeGrue, S. J. and Hearn, D. R., Extraction of immunogenic and suppressogenic antigens from variants of B16 melanoma exhibiting low or high metastatic potentials, *Cancer Res.*, 43, 5106, 1983.
25. Miller, F. R., Concomitant tumor immunity in the mammary gland, *Cancer Immunol. Immunother.*, 20, 219, 1985.

26. Miller, F. R., Miller, B. E., and Heppner, G. H., Characterization of metastatic heterogeneity among subpopulations of a single mouse mammary tumor: heterogeneity in phenotypic stability, *Invasion Met.,* 3, 22, 1983.

27. Miller, B. E., Miller, F. R., Leith, J. and Heppner, G. H., Growth interaction *in vivo* between tumor subpopulations derived from a single mouse mammary tumor, *Cancer Res.,* 40, 3977, 1980.

28. Rios, A. M., Miller, F. R., and Heppner, G. H., Characterization of tumor-associated lymphocytes in a series of mouse mammary tumor lines with differing biological properties, *Cancer Immunol. Immunother.,* 15, 87, 1983.

29. Mahoney, K. H., Fulton, A. M., and Heppner, G. H., Tumor-associated macrophages of mouse mammary tumors. II. Differential distribution of macrophages from metastatic and nonmetastatic tumors, *J. Immunol.,* 131, 2079, 1983.

30. Mahoney, K. H., Miller, B. E., and Heppner, G. H., FACs quantitation of leucine aminopeptidase and acid phosphatase on tumor-associated macrophages from metastatic and nonmetastatic mouse mammary tumors, *J. Leukocyte Biol.,* 38, 573, 1985.

31. Schirrmacher, V., Bosslet, K., Shantz, G., Clauer, K., and Hubsch, D., Tumor metastases and cell-mediated immunity in a model system in DBA/2 mice. IV. Antigenic differences between a metastasizing variant and the parental tumor line revealed by cytotoxic T lymphocytes, *Int. J. Cancer,* 23, 245, 1979.

32. Bosslet, K., Schirrmacher, V., and Shantz, G., Tumor metastases and cell-mediated immunity in a model system in DBA/2 mice. VI. Similar specificity patterns of protective anti-tumor immunity *in vivo* and of cytolytic T cells *in vitro, Int. J. Cancer,* 24, 303, 1979.

33. Fogel, M., Altevogt, P., and Schirrmacher, V., Metastatic potential severely altered by changes in tumor cell adhesiveness and cell surface sialylation, *J. Exp. Med.,* 157, 371, 1983.

34. Altevogt, P., Fogel, M., Cheingsong-Popov, R., Dennis, J., Robinson, P., and Schirrmacher, V., Different patterns of lectin binding and cell surface sialylation detected on related high- and low-metastatic tumor lines, *Cancer Res.,* 43, 5138, 1983.

35. Simmons, R. L. and Rios, A., Differential effect of neuraminidase on the immunogenicity of viral associated and private antigens of mammary carcinomas, *J. Immunol.,* 111, 1820, 1973.

36. Tao, T.-W. and Burger, M. M., Lectin-resistant variants of mouse melanoma cells. I. Altered metastasizing capacity and tumorigenicity, *Int. J. Cancer,* 29, 425, 1982.

37. Reading, C. L., Brunson, K. W., Torrianni, M., and Nicolson, G. L., Malignancies of metastatic murine lymphosarcoma cell lines and clones correlate with decreased cell surface display of RNA tumor virus envelope glycoprotein gp70, in *Proc. Natl. Acad. Sci. U.S.A.,* 77, 5943, 1980.

38. Kumar, R. K., Price, J. E., Sargent, N. S. E., and Tarin, D., Binding of ^{125}I-labelled Concanavalian A by cells from spontaneously arising murine mammary carcinomas and experimentally induced metastases, *Anticancer Res.,* 3, 343, 1983.

39. Hagmar, B. and Ryd, W., Altered experimental metastasis pattern by proteolytic cell treatment, *Invasion Met.,* 5, 31, 1985.

40. Shearman, P. J. and Longenecker, B. M., Clonal variation and functional correlation of organ-specific metastasis and an organ-specific metastasis-associated antigen, *Int. J. Cancer,* 27, 387, 1981.

41. Shearman, P. J., Gallatin, W. M., and Longenecker, B. M., Detection of a cell-surface antigen correlated with organ-specific metastasis, *Nature (London),* 286, 267, 1980.

42. Fidler, I. J., Gersten, D. M., and Budmen, M. B., Characterization *in vivo* and *in vitro* of tumor cells selected for resistance to syngeneic lymphocyte-mediated cytotoxicity, *Cancer Res.,* 36, 3160, 1976.

43. Bosslet, K. and Schirrmacher, V., High-frequency generation of new immunoresistant tumor variants during metastasis of a cloned murine tumor line (ESb), *Int. J. Cancer,* 29, 195, 1982.

44. Bosslet, K. and Schirrmacher, V., Escape of metastasizing clonal tumor cell variants from tumor-specific cytolytic T lymphocytes, *J. Exp. Med.,* 154, 557, 1981.

45. Katzav, S., Segal, S., and Feldman, M., Immuno-selection *in vivo* of H-2D phenotypic variants from a metastatic clone of sarcoma cells results in cell lines of altered metastatic competence, *Int. J. Cancer,* 33, 407, 1984.

46. DeBaetselier, P., Katzav, S., Gorelik, E., Feldman, M., and Segal, S., Differential expression of H-2 gene products in tumour cells is associated with their metastatogenic properties, *Nature (London),* 288, 179, 1980.

47. Eisenbach, L., Segal, S., and Feldman, M., MHC imbalance and metastatic spread in Lewis lung carcinoma clones, *Int. J. Cancer,* 32, 113, 1983.

48. Eisenbach, L., Hollander, N., Greenfield, L., Yakor, H., Segal, S., and Feldman, M., The differential expression of H-2K versus H-2D antigens, distinguishing high-metastatic from low-metastatic clones, is correlated with the immunogenic properties of the tumor cells, *Int. J. Cancer,* 34, 567, 1984.

49. Nowotny, A. and Grohsman, J., Mixed tumor challenge of strain specific and nonspecific TA3 mouse ascites mammary adenocarcinoma, *Int. Arch. Allergy,* 44, 434, 1973.

50. Georlette, M. and Boon, T., Immunogenic cell variants of a mouse teratocarcinoma confer a protection against the original non-immunogenic transplantable tumor, *Eur. J. Cancer Clin. Oncol.,* 17, 1083, 1981.
51. Miller, F. R. and Heppner, G. H., Immunologic heterogeneity of tumor cell subpopulations from a single mouse mammary tumor, *J. Natl. Cancer Inst.,* 63, 1457, 1979.
52. Prehn, R. T., Analysis of antigenic heterogeneity within individual 3-methylcholanthrane-induced mouse sarcomas, *J. Natl. Cancer Inst.,* 45, 1039, 1970.
53. Urban, J. L., Van Waes, C., and Schreiber, H., Pecking order among tumor-specific antigens, *Eur. J. Immunol.,* 14, 181, 1984.
54. Miller, F. R., Tumor subpopulation interactions in metastasis, *Invasion Met.,* 3, 234, 1983.
55. Miller, F. R., Verification of subpopulation interactions in experimental metastasis with genetic markers, in *Proc. Am. Assoc. Cancer Res.,* 25, 53 (Abstr.), 1984.
56. Cikes, M., Friberg, S., Jr., and Klein, G., Quantitative studies of antigen expression in cultured murine lymphoma cells. II. Cell-surface antigens in synchronized cultures, *J. Natl. Cancer Inst.,* 49, 1607, 1972.
57. Lerner, R. A., Oldstone, M. B. A., and Cooper, N. R., Cell cycle-dependent immune lysis of Moloney virus-transformed lymphocytes: presence of viral antigen, accessibility to antibody, and complement activation, in *Proc. Natl. Acad. Sci. U.S.A.,* 68, 2584, 1971.
58. Pasternak, C. A., Warmsley, A. M. H., and Thomas, D. B., Structural alterations in the surface membrane during the cell cycle, *J. Cell Biol.,* 50, 562, 1971.
59. Suzuki, N., Frapart, M., Grdina, D. J., Meistrich, M. L., and Withers, H. R., Cell cycle dependency of metastatic lung colony formation, *Cancer Res.,* 37, 3690, 1977.
60. Bahler, D. W., Lord, E. M., Kennel, S. J., and Horan, P. K., Heterogeneity and clonal variation related to cell surface expression of a mouse lung tumor-associated antigen quantified using flow cytometry, *Cancer Res.,* 144, 3317, 1984.
61. Taupier, M. A., Kearney, J. F., Leibson, P. J., Loken, M. R., and Schreiber, H., Nonrandom escape of tumor cells from immune lysis due to intraclonal fluctuations in antigen expression, *Cancer Res.,* 43, 4050, 1983.
62. Shapiro, S. J., Leibson, P. J., Loken, M. R., and Schreiber, H., Changes in susceptibility to cytotoxic antibody among tumor cells surviving exposure to chemotherapeutic agents, *Cancer Res.,* 42, 2622, 1982.
63. Greiner, J. W., Horan Hand, P., Noguchi, P., Fisher, P. B., Pestka, S., and Schlom, J., Enhanced expression of surface tumor-associated antigens on human breast and colon tumor cells after recombinant human leukocyte α-interferon treatment, *Cancer Res.,* 44, 3208, 1984.
64. Poste, G., Doll, J., and Fidler, I. J., Interactions among clonal subpopulations affect stability of the metastatic phenotype in polyclonal populations of B16 melanoma cells, in *Proc. Natl. Acad. Sci. U.S.A.,* 78, 6226, 1981.
65. Harris, J. F., Chambers, A. F., Hill, R. P., and Ling, V., Metastatic variants are generated spontaneously at a high rate in mouse KHT tumor, in *Proc. Natl. Acad. Sci. U.S.A.,* 79, 5547, 1982.
66. Neri, A. and Nicolson, G. L., Phenotypic drift of metastatic and cell-surface properties of mammary adenocarcinoma cell clones during growth, *in vitro, Int. J. Cancer,* 28, 731, 1981.
67. Goldie, J. H. and Coldman, A. J., The genetic origin of drug resistance in neoplasms: implications for systemic therapy, *Cancer Res.,* 44, 3643, 1984.

Chapter 3

MHC ANTIGEN EXPRESSION AND METASTATIC PROPERTIES OF TUMOR CELLS

Elieser Gorelik

TABLE OF CONTENTS

I. INTRODUCTION

Metastasis formation is a multistep, highly selective process. Tumor cells are constantly released into the blood circulation during local tumor growth. Detection of even 1 malignant cell per mm^3 of blood is equivalent to the constant presence of approximately 5×10^6 cells in the blood of a 70 kg man.[1] However, it is widely agreed that the detection of tumor cells in the circulation has no prognostic significance.[2] The incidence and the number of the metastatic foci which can be found at autopsy is considerably lower than the potential number which might be expected from the presence of numerous cancer cells in the circulation. Entering of tumor cells into the blood stream is just the initial step in the metastatic cascade and not sufficient for the apparent metastatic growth. Using a method of i.v. inoculation of the radiolabeled tumor cells, it was determined that only a small proportion (about 0.1%) of inoculated tumor cells are able to form metastatic foci in the lungs.[3]

The relatively low yield of metastatic tumors in comparison to tumor cells spreading in the body could be attributed to at least two major reasons: (1) some tumor cells lack the properties required to fulfill the metastatic cascade, and (2) although some tumor cells possess all these properties, they, in addition, have some characteristic which allow the host's resistance mechanisms to interfere with the realization of their potential metastatic ability.

Numerous studies were conducted to characterize the metastatic phenotype of tumor cells. Most of these studies were performed by comparison of proteins, glycoproteins, glycolipids, enzyme production, biophysical, and adhesive parameters, as well as the invasive properties of tumor cells with low and high metastatic potency (for reviews, see References 4 to 7). Although the results of these investigations do not precisely define what tumor cell properties are required for metastatic spread, it appears that only a certain portion of tumor cell population possesses the characteristics which are required for extravasation, invasion, and proliferation in a new environment. In addition, the realization of the metastatic potential of tumor cells largely depends on their ability to escape the elimination by the host defense mechanisms.

An increasing body of evidence indicates that immune mechanisms could play an important role in the destruction of metastatic cells. Some experimental tumors failed to develop metastatic tumors in the immunocompetent host, but they become metastatic in the immunosuppressed or immunodeficient animals.[8-12] The level of the immunogenicity of tumor cells varies over a wide range. Using high, middle, and nonimmunogenic tumors, Fidler et al.[12] have shown that metastasis formation by highly immunogenic tumor cells was dramatically increased in immunosuppressed mice, whereas such augmentation of growth was less profound for the less immunogenic tumor cells.

Metastasis formation takes place despite the presence of immune reactions which develop against the locally growing tumor cells. Most migrating potentially metastatic tumor cells could be eliminated by such immune reactions and just cells which could resist this immune attack have the potential to form metastatic foci in distant anatomical locations. Recent data indicate that, in addition to specific T-cell immunity, natural cell-mediated immunity also participates in the control of metastatic spread and growth.[43 45,47,51] NK cells and macrophages could eliminate tumor cells regardless of their immunogenicity. For nonimmunogenic tumors these effector cells represent the main line in the antimetastatic defense.[43-45,47,51] Therefore, immunoselection could be due in part to the selection forces involved in the formation of the phenotype of the metastatic cell population.

II. ANTIGENIC HETEROGENEITY OF TUMOR CELLS

A tumor is a heterogeneous population of malignant cells, composed of a series of related but phenotypically distinct individual clones. Morphological divergency of the malignant cells was well documented many years ago during pathohistological examination of malignant tumors. The development of techniques for chromosomal analysis of normal and malignant cells[13] revealed consistent chromosomal composition in normal tissue but striking heterogeneity in the number and structure of the chromosomes among malignant cells. Intensive studies of tumor cell cytogenetics resulted in the formation of the stem-line concept.[14-16] According to this hypothesis, a tumor cell population contains a predominant clone (stem-line) and numerous sideline clones. Some tumors have two or more stem lines. Genotypic heterogeneity of tumor cell populations provides a high level of plasticity and adaptation to the environment.[16,17] Although tumor cells are characterized by relatively high levels of chromosomal and gene mutability,[18,19] the genotypes of the tumor cell populations are not "shiftless drifters in a state of neoplastic anarchy".[16] Specific tumor karyotypes have competitive survival value and will be constant for thousands of cell generations if the environment permits.[16]

Genetic clonal heterogeneity of tumor cell populations is the basis of their heterogeneity in many phenotypic characteristics such as biochemical properties, drug and radiation sensitivity, degree of malignancy, invasiveness and metastatic ability, and their antigenic and immunogenic properties (see reviews in References 4, 20 to 22).

Recently, it was suggested that epigenetic mechanisms could also contribute to the diversification of tumor cell properties.[23] Upon exposure to toxic treatments (chemotherapeutic drugs, irradiation, immune attack) some tumor clones are eliminated but others escape lethal damage and propagate. Thus, tumor cell heterogeneity might be one of the obstacles responsible for the failure of different therapeutic modalities to cure malignant disease.

Based on karyotypic shifts of tumor cell populations when transplanted into mice across allogeneic barriers, the existance of antigenic heterogeneity was suggested, with immunoselection playing a role in the determination of the phenotypic profile of the tumor cell population.[16,24,25] Antigenic heterogeneity within methylcholanthrene (MC)-induced tumor was first demonstrated by Prehn[26] using immunization and challenge with tumor lines derived from different fragments taken from opposite sides of the same MC-induced sarcoma. By cloning various rodent tumors, heterogeneity and antigenic specificity of the individual clones was demonstrated.[21,23,27,30]

The significance of the immunogenic and antigenic heterogeneity of tumor cell populations can be illustrated by the following experiments. Spleen cells or serum of mice bearing Ehrlich carcinoma or NK/Ly lymphoma were able to inhibit tumor growth and shift the karyotypic profile of these tumors.[28,29] As a result of exposure of the tumor cells to serum and complement, tumor variants arose which were resistant to the initially cytotoxic serum. In addition, they lost hyperdiploid and some triploid cell clones and a new tetraploid clone become predominant in these populations.[29] The resistance of new tumor sublines to complement-dependent cytolysis was not due to the selection of antigen loss variants, but mostly to the selection of clones with different antigenic specificities. Indeed, resistant variants of Ehrlich carcinoma or NK/Ly lymphoma were able to induce immune responses after transplantation into new host and sera of mice bearing these "resistant" sublines were highly cytotoxic against "resistant" tumor variants but only partially active against the parental tumors.[29] Based on these findings, it was proposed that during tumor growth immune responses evoked against each clone and are primarily directed against the most immunogenic clones. As a result of immune attack, these immunogenic clones could be eliminated or their growth could be inhibited, whereas other clones would be undamaged and expand. Thus, antigenic and immunogenic heterogeneity of tumor cell populations could be a factor which helps a tumor to escape immune destruction.[29]

Additional experimental support for this assumption came from investigations performed by Olsson and Ebbesen.[30] They found that thymomas of AKR mice consist of a predominant clone (97% cells) plus three antigenically distinctive clones, representing just 3% of the whole tumor cell population. By immunization with irradiated thymoma cells, antitumor resistance could be induced only in 30% of immunized mice. The tumors which arose in the rest of immunized mice were antigenically distinct from the original tumor. This could be attributed to the preferential focus of the immune response on the predominant clone, with other clones able to grow. When immunization procedures included a mixture of equal numbers of cells from each clone, there was a dramatic increase in the efficiency of specific immunization and antitumor resistance against the original thymoma was induced in more than 90% of immunized mice.[30]

Using various experimental tumors, it was demonstrated that animals, after surgical excision of the local tumor, became immune to the second tumor challenge.[26] It is conceivable that growth of residual tumor cells in the operated animals also prevented by immune mechanisms. However, as discussed above for other tumors, clones with different antigenic specificity may have a better chance to survive and develop new tumors. Indeed, Pimm and Baldwin[31] have found that recurrent tumors were immunologically distinct from the original resected primary tumor.

In fact, for some tumor systems, it was demonstrated that immune attack by the host resulted in the selection of nonimmunogenic antigen loss tumor cell variants.[11,32,33]

Recent success in the development of monoclonal antibodies provides a powerful tool for the further analysis of the antigenic heterogeneity of tumor cell populations. Using monoclonal antibodies, antigenic heterogeneity of human tumors of various histological origins was clearly demonstrated.[34-36]

Thus, antigenic heterogeneity and immunoselection of nonimmunogenic clones or clones with different antigenic specificities could be an important mechanisms of escape of tumor cells from the host's immune reactions and could be the major mechanisms responsible for the failures of therapy with monoclonal antibodies or of specific immunotherapy.

III. IMMUNOSELECTION AND FORMATION OF METASTATIC TUMOR CELL POPULATION

A. Antigenic Differences Between Primary and Metastatic Tumor Cells

Since the metastatic process occurs at the time when the immune response is developed against primary tumors growing locally, it is expected that metastatic tumor cells, which can escape immune destruction, have a chance to survive and further develop metastatic tumors. This prediction is attributed to the tumors which are able to induce a specific immune response. Based on this assumption, it is expected that metastatic cells might be nonimmunogenic, nonantigenic, or display antigenic specificities which differ from the primary tumor cells.

During the last 10 years, intensive studies of the comparative antigenic profile of tumor cells from primary and metastatic sites were performed. Technically, these studies included immunization-challenge with primary or metastatic tumor cells, or assessment of the sensitivity of tumor cells to the specific immune lymphocytes or of their ability to bind specific monoclonal antibodies.

Deichman and Kluchareva[33] were probably the first to demonstrate that immunogenic hamster SV-40-induced tumor cells were able to metastasize only after losing their antigenicity.

Sugarbaker and Cohen[37] compared the immunogenic and antigenic characteristics of tumor cells derived from the primary (P) murine sarcoma and from 7 individual pulmonary metastatic foci. The results of this study can be summarized as follows: three metastatic (M) tumor lines (M2, M6, and M9), in comparison to the P tumor, showed distinctive antigenic and immunogenic properties. Two metastatic lines (M10 and M15) were nonimmunogenic and nonantigenic since they failed to induce immune resistance against themselves or against P tumor cells. In addition, immunization with P tumor cells did not affect the growth of M10 or M15 cells. Two other metastatic lines (M13 and M16) had shared common antigenic and immunogenic characteristics with P tumor. They immunized mice against themselves and against P and vice versa.

Antigenic differences between locally growing 3LL (L-3LL) and its pulmonary metastasis (M-3LL) were found when normal spleen cells were sensitized in vitro against these tumor lines.[38,39] Spleen cells immunized against L-3LL were preferentially cytotoxic against L-3LL but less against M-3LL tumor cells. Similarly, spleen cells immune against M-3LL showed higher cytotoxic activity against M-3LL than L-3LL target. When L-3LL and M-3LL tumor cells were admixed with immune spleen cells and inoculated into the footpads of syngeneic mice, spleen cells immune against M-3LL, but not against L-3LL, significantly inhibited the formation of the metastatic foci in mice bearing L-3LL or M-3LL tumors.[38,39]

The antigenic specificity of the rat primary MC-induced sarcoma and its metastasis was investigated by Pimm et al.[40] Using cross-immunization of rats with primary tumor or tumor lines derived from metastases into lungs, kidney, or peritoneum, it was found that primary tumor cells and tumor cells from peritoneal metastases shared common antigens, whereas metastatic cells from the lung or kidney had distinctive antigenic specificities. Metastatic cells from the lung or kidney were able to induce protection against each other, but not against peritoneal metastatic cells.[40]

The existance of antigenic diversity between human metastatic and primary tumors was also observed. Using a battery of monoclonal antibodies directed against various melanoma antigens, Albino et al.[34] found antigenic differences among individual metastases in the same patient with malignant melanoma. Furthermore, the autologous serum of this patient contained antibodies which reacted with only one, but not the other six, metastatic tumor lines.[34] Using monoclonal antibodies to carcinoembryonic antigen (CEA), it was found that metastases in patients with highly CEA-positive primary colon carcinoma could be CEA-negative, and CEA-positive metastases could be found when the primary tumors were CEA-negative.[35]

Similarly, diversity in the binding of monoclonal antibodies by primary vs. metastatic tumor cells was observed in most of 15 human sarcomas investigated.[36]

Although antigenic and immunogenic differences between primary and metastatic tumor cells have been demonstrated, it is impossible to extrapolate these data to all metastatic tumors. Since some tumors are nonimmunogenic, the metastatic tumor cells would not be a target for specific immune reactions and antigenic diversity between primary and metastatic tumors would not be expected. In addition, the level of immunoselective pressure should be taken into consideration when results of antigenicity and immunogenicity of metastatic cells are analyzed. The antitumor immune response in tumor-bearing animals usually has biphasic characteristics: after the initial response, immunologic reactivity usually declines as the tumor mass increases.[41,42] In contrast, the number of tumor cells shed into the blood proportionally increases with an increase in the volume of the primary tumor.[4] Thus, under these conditions, the immunoselective pressure declines and more tumor cells have the potential to survive and develop metastatic tumors, regardless of their antigenic and immunogenic properties. This could also serve as an explanation for the frequent observation that there is similarity between primary tumor cells and tumor cells derived from some individual metastatic foci, whereas other foci are antigenically distinctive. Although malignant tumors can be weakly or nonimmunogenic and lack the ability to induce detectable T-cell-mediated immunity, their metastatic tumor could be the target for immunoselection mediated by other immune effector mechanisms.

Recent experimental data indicate that, in addition to or as an alternative to specific T-lymphocytes, NK cells and/or activated macrophages might be tumoricidal and participate in the immunoselection of the tumor cell population during metastasis formation.

B. NK Cells and Metastatic Growth

It was found that NK cells play an important role in the intravascular elimination of tumor cells and in the control of metastatic spread.[43-47] This conclusion was based on the following findings:

1. Elimination of the radiolabeled tumor cells after i.v. inoculation positively correlated with the level of NK reactivity in the recipients. Nude mice with high levels of NK cell activity were more efficient for tumor cell elimination than mice of strains with lower NK reactivity.[43-47] Beige mice or very young mice (3-weeks-old), which have low levels of NK reactivity, showed relatively high survival of i.v. inoculated tumor cells and more metastatic foci developed in the lungs of these mice.[43,45]

2. NK cell function has been depressed by pretreatment of mice with irradiation, cyclophosphamide, β-estradiol, corticosteroids, urethane, anti-asialo GM-1 serum, or NK 1.1 or NK 1.2 antiserum. Treatment of mice with these agents resulted in depression of tumor cell elimination, and in increased formation of experimental or spontaneous tumor foci in the lungs.[43-51]

   It is of interest that in mice with depressed NK reactivity, i.e., beige mice or mice after treatment with cyclophosphamide or anti-asialo GM-1 serum, the dramatic increases in the number of the pulmonary B16 melanoma metastases were accompanied by increased formation of extrapulmonary, especially liver, metastases which rarely occur, if at all, in mice with normal NK reactivity.[43,44,50] These data indicate the B16 melanoma cells have the inherent ability to settle and proliferate in the liver, but ordinarily, their growth is efficiently prevented by NK cells.

3. The cytotoxic activity of NK cells can be stimulated by pretreatment of mice with *Corynebacterium parvum,* BCG, and poly I:C. In parallel, treatment of mice with these agents was found to be associated with an increase in the clearance of radiolabeled tumor cells from the pulmonary vasculature and a decrease in the number of the detectable experimental or spontaneous metastases.[45,48,50]

4. More direct evidence for the involvement of NK cells in intravascular tumor cell destruction and inhibition of metastasis formation has come from experiments with adoptively transferred NK-enriched or depleted lymphoid cell populations. NK reactivity of mice depressed by cyclophosphamide (Cy) or anti-asialo GM-1 treatment could be reconstituted by adoptive transfer of lymphoid cells. In parallel, adoptively transferred lymphoid cells were able to reconstitute the antimetastatic resistance of these mice.[43,53] Spleen cells with depleted NK cell activity failed to restore antimetastatic defenses in the NK-suppressed recipients.[43,53] Similar results were obtained when NK reactivity and antimetastatic resistance of rats treated with anti-asialo GM-1 serum were reconstituted by transfusion highly purified syngeneic large granular lymphocytes.[54]

These experimental data strongly support the concept that NK cells can be extremely efficient in the intravascular elimination of tumor cells and in prevention of metastasis formation, although it is impossible to exclude the involvement in these processes of additional cells such as neutrophils, monocytes, or of humoral factors such as natural antibodies or complement.[55,56]

Since NK cells could participate in the elimination of tumor cells from the blood, one might predict that tumor cells which survive and successfully metastasize would be more resistant to lysis by NK cells than tumor cells derived from local sites of tumor growth. Indeed, in our previous experiments, when the cytotoxic activity of normal spleen cells was tested against 3LL tumor cells derived from the local tumor or from spontaneous pulmonary metastases, higher resistance was found among metastatic cells.[57] Furthermore, serial subcutaneous transfer of 3LL tumor cells mixed with normal spleen cells in a ratio of 1:100 resulted in the selection of tumor cells displaying both higher resistance to the cytotoxic action of NK cells and higher metastatic ability.[58,59]

In analogous studies of rat spontaneous mammary adenocarcinoma and their metastases,[60] tumor cells derived from the pulmonary or lymph node metastases, as well as from pleural effusions, were also found to be more resistant to NK activity. The resistance of metastatic cells to NK cells was observed when the tumor cells were isolated directly from the metastatic nodules, but this resistance disappeared after in vitro propagation.[60]

In additional experiments, metastatic cells derived from two lung foci and tumor cells from the primary hamster histiocytic tumor were compared for their susceptibility to NK activity.[61] The parental tumor cells were weakly metastatic and highly susceptible to the cytotoxic action of normal blood lymphocytes or spleen cells. In contrast, tumor cells derived from metastatic nodules in the lungs were highly metastatic and exhibited high levels of resistance to NK mediated cytotoxicity.[61]

In all of the above experiments, resistance to lysis by NK cells was demonstrated when tumor cells were derived from spontaneous metastases. In contrast, when the susceptibility or resistance of tumor cells to NK activity were compared with their ability to develop artificial metastatic nodules after i.v. inoculation, rather divergent results were observed. B16 melanoma sublines (B16F1, B16F10, and B16F10^{Lr}) vary in their lung colonizing potential but have similar levels of susceptibility to NK cell-mediated cytotoxicity.[62] Furthermore, no correlation was found between the number of pulmonary experimental metastases developed by clones selected from K-1735 melanoma or UV-2237 fibrosarcoma and the susceptibility of the investigated clones to cytotoxic activity of NK cells.[62] However, the importance of NK resistance for metastatic potential was demonstrated when the metastatic properties of tumor cells were compared in nude mice, which are characterized by relatively high levels of NK reactivity.[62] Repeated incubation of UV-2237 tumor cells with nylon-wool-nonadherent spleen cells resulted in the selection of tumor cell variants which expressed high levels of resistance to NK-mediated cytotoxicity and high metastatic properties in nude mice. The differences in the metastatic potential between sensitive and resistant tumor cells lines was not observed when these lines were inoculated into 3-week-old nude mice with relatively low NK reactivity.[62] Thus, the metastatic advantage of NK-resistant tumor cells was observed only in mice with relatively high NK reactivity. This conclusion is also supported by experiments in which NK sensitivity and metastatsis formation of various clones of 3LL tumor was compared. NK-resistant clones, after i.v. inoculation, developed more metastatic foci in the lungs than NK-sensitive clones. However, no differences in the number of metastases was found when NK-resistant and NK-sensitive 3LL clones were inoculated into beige mice.[63]

In general, although some experimental data indicate that NK resistance could be an important component of the metastatic phenotype, NK resistance cannot completely account for the ability of tumor cells to metastasize. Metastatic cells have to possess a complex series of properties which allow them to fulfill the entire sequence of steps involved in the metastatic cascade.

C. Macrophages and Metastasis Formation

An increasing body of experimental data indicates that, in addition to T- and NK-cells, macrophages could participate in the control of metastatic process.[65-68,70]

Activated macrophages exert in vitro a high level of cytotoxic and cytostatic activity against a variety of tumor cells.[64,69] Although selection of tumor cells which are completely resistant to the tumoricidal effects of macrophage is less common than selection of resistance to T- and NK-cells,[62] heterogeneity of tumor cells in sensitivity to lysis by activated macrophages was documented in numerous investigations.[65-67,71,72] The positive correlation between metastatic properties of tumor cells and their resistance to the tumoricidal action of activated macrophages, is at least suggestive evidence for the involvement of macrophages in the elimination of potentially metastatic tumor cells.

The first in vivo evidence of the possible involvement of macrophages in the control of metastatic spread were obtained when the metastatic properties of cloned and uncloned population of murine RAW 117 lymphosarcoma were investigated.[73] It was demonstrated that sublines or individual clones of RAW 117 lymphosarcoma which were able to develop liver metastasis were characterized by low levels of gp70 expression. The original lymphosarcoma or its clones with high gp70 expression on cell membranes failed to colonize the liver in normal or nude mice. Suppression of NK cell function in these mice had no effect on antimetastatic resistance. Only when mice were treated with silica or carrageenan agents which suppressed macrophage function, RAW 117 lymphosarcoma cells were able to form metastases in the liver.[74] In addition, a comparison of the susceptibility of metastatic and nonmetastatic RAW 117 sublines and clones to cytotoxic and cytostatic action of activated peritoneal macrophages revealed that high metastatic potential positively correlated with high resistance to the cytostatic and cytotoxic effects of macrophages.[66]

A similar association between the relative resistance to the tumoricidal action of activated macrophages and high metastatic performance was also demonstrated with other experimental tumors such as a chemically induced murine sarcoma,[68] a spontaneous mammary adenocarcinoma,[67] the B16 melanoma and its highly metastatic sublines B16-B14b,[65] and metastatic and nonmetastatic sublines of the mammary adenocarcinoma 13762NF.[75]

It is of interest that differences in sensitivity or resistance to the tumoricidal activity of activated macrophages were found only with tumor cells, were isolated from in vivo growing tumors and no differences in sensitivity were observed when tumor cells were tested after in vitro culture.[75] Similar findings were obtained when the NK sensitivity of tumor cells isolated from primary and metastatic tumors were tested.[40]

IV. MHC ANTIGEN EXPRESSION BY TUMOR CELLS

Major histocompatibility complex (MHC) gene products play an important role in the stimulation and regulation of specific T-cell-mediated immunity. Immune lymphocytes recognize foreign antigens in association with MHC antigens.[76] Elimination of tumor cells by specific immune mechanisms appears to require the expression of class I MHC molecules and TATA.[76] Tumor cells could be nonimmunogenic as a result of the lack or diminished expression of either the MHC antigens and/or TATA.

Direct analysis of the cell surface spontaneous and induced murine tumors for expression of H-2 antigens using polyclonal or monoclonal antibodies revealed numerous quantitative and qualitative alterations in the expression of class I antigens of H-2 complex.[76-78] Similar investigations performed on tumors of cancer patients demonstrated that in many human tumors, HLA antigens remained undetectable or their expression was severely diminished. Almost 50% of investigated melanomas, breast carcinomas, skin carcinomas, and neuroblastomas had various changes in expression of HLA-A,B,C antigens or β_2-microglobulin.[79-82] Of the 11 investigated human small-cell lung cancer (SCLC) 10 cell lines did not express at all or expressed low levels of β_2-microglobulin and class I HLA antigens.

In contrast, almost all investigated nonsmall-cell lung cancer (NSCLC) cell lines had high level of expression of β_2-microglobulin and HLA-A,B,C antigens.[82] SCLC cells in parallel with lack of MHC antigens exhibited rapid growth and early metastases. The degree of malignancy for SCLC cells was also associated with an amplification of the c-myc oncogene. It is of interest that SCLC cell lines with the greatest level of c-myc amplification had the lowest level of MHC antigen expression.[82] In accordance with these findings, neuroblastoma cell lines which had amplification of the N-myc oncogene also demonstrated a high incidence of alteration of MHC gene expression.[80] It was suggested that down regulation of MHC genes can be a common aspect of malignant transformation mediated by oncogenes.[82] An inverse relationship between expression of MHC class I antigen and degree of malignancy was also demonstrated for some other human tumors. Eccrine porocarcinomas of the skin exist in benign and malignant forms and histological discrimination not always possible. It was found that malignant porocarcinomas completely lost β_2-microglobulin and HLA class I antigens whereas benign tumors fully express these antigens.[81]

These alterations in MHC antigen expression on the tumor cell surface are probably not accidental and might provide them with the possibility to escape immune destruction. Recently, this assumption has received strong experimental support.

C3H fibroblasts were transformed in vitro with SV-40 virus and adapted to grow in vivo. Most of transformed clones failed to grow in the immunocompetent syngeneic mice if they fully expressed the H-2 antigens. Tumor cells, which were able to grow in mice, did not express H-2K^k antigens.[84]

Rat or murine tumor cells transformed by human adenovirus type 12 did not express MHC class I antigens and were tumorigenic. In contrast, malignant cells transformed with adenovirus type 5 expressed MHC antigens and were rejected in the immunocompetent syngeneic host.[85,86]

The importance of MHC antigen for tumor cell immunogenicity was supported by the results of H-2 gene transfection experiments. After H-2 gene transfection, H-2-negative adenovirus type 12 transformed murine tumor cells became H-2-positive and also appeared to be highly immunogenic, since they were rejected in the immunocompetent mice.[86]

AKR lymphoma cells which lost H-2K^k antigens were nonimmunogenic and highly tumorigenic.[77] Immunogenicity of this AKR lymphoma was completely reconstituted following transfection of the H-2K^k gene.[87]

These experiments demonstrate that failure of the immune system to react against H-2-negative tumor cells is not due to the absence of TATA, but rather to the absence of MHC-restricted molecules.

A. MHC Antigens and Metastatic Growth

Changes in MHC expression might confer certain advantages to potentially metastatic cells and provide them with the possibility to form metastatic foci in different anatomic locations, even when an immune response has been evoked by the primary tumor mass. Thus, the observed antigenic differences between primary and metastatic tumor cells could be a result of differences in the expression of TATA and/or class I MHC antigens.

The first attempts to compare histocompatibility antigens on the cell surface of tumor cells from primary and metastatic tumors were reported by Axelrad and Klein.[88] The level of expression of the histocompatability antigens by the primary and metastatic tumor cells was evaluated by their ability to grow in allogeneic F2 hybrid mice.

There were two types of the primary tumors and metastases tested: tumor spontaneously originated in (A/StK1 × C3H/StK1) F1 mice or in the parental strain C3H/StK1. The results of testing the ability of the primary and metastatic tumors to grow in F2 hybrids indicated that metastases from F1 tumors had a significantly lower incidence of takes in F2 mice than primary F1 tumor. On the contrary, metastases from the tumor which originated in homozygous C3H mice grew more successfully in F2 mice than did those from the primary tumor.[88]

A comparison of tumor cells derived from lymph node metastases with those from a primary spontaneous mammary adenocarcinoma of C3H/DiSn mice (H-2^k haplotype) revealed that the metastatic tumor cells had different karyotypic characteristics, were able to grow in ascites form after i.p. transplantation and developed progressively growing tumors in allogeneic Af (H-2^a) and C57BL/6 (H-2^b) mice. In contrast, growth of tumor cells from the primary spontaneous mammary adenocarcinoma in allogeneic mice was completely prevented.[89]

Haywood and McKhann[99] investigated the relationship between H-2 antigen expression, immunogenicity, and metastatic ability using five MC-induced tumors of C3H/HeJ origin. Tumor cell H-2 antigen expression was assessed by quantitative absorption of anti-H-2 serum with tumor cells. Tumor cells with relatively high expression of H-2 antigens had relatively low level of TATA expression (tested by immunization and secondary challange). In contrast, more immunogenic tumors had lower H-2 class I antigen expression.[90] High metastatic ability was detected in mice bearing tumors which had H-2 high and TATA low expression. Less metastatic cells were in the lungs when tumors had relatively low H-2 and high TATA expression.[90]

During our investigation of the antigenic profiles of primary L-3LL and metastasis-derived M-3LL tumor cells, we found that M-3LL tumor cells had a higher incidence of takes in allogeneic mice than did L-3LL cells. Although 3LL cells were able to grow locally in some allogeneic mice, they failed to develop distant metastases.[91] These findings stimulated further investigations of the expression of H-2 antigens on the cell surface of the L-3LL and M-3LL tumor cells using polyclonal and monoclonal antibodies and analysis of flow cytometry. It was found that L-3LL tumor cells express relatively low levels of H-2K^b antigens and relatively high levels of H-2D^b antigens.[40,92 94] In the line of these findings anti-H-2D^b, but not anti-H-2K^b, CTL were cytotoxic against 3LL tumor cells. Immunization of allogenic mice with 3LL tumor cells resulted in production of mostly anti-H-2D^b antibodies.[92,93] Thus, the ability of 3LL tumor cells to grow across of allogenic barrier appeared to be due to disproportional expression of H-2K^b and H-2D^b molecules.

Using allogenic and congenic strains of mice, it was demonstrated that locally growing 3LL tumor cells developed spontaneous pulmonary metastatic tumors in mice which shared H-2D^b antigens and the C57BL/6 genetic background (minor histocompatibility antigens).[92] Macroscopic pulmonary metastases did not develop in BALB/c mice bearing allogeneic 3LL tumors. By transfer of the lungs of BALB/c mice bearing 3LL tumor into (BALB/c × C57BL/6) F1 mice, it was found that tumor cells were shed and migrate into the lungs but their growth was arrested by immune mechanisms. Indeed, in the immunosuppressed or athymic nude allogeneic mice 3LL tumors grew locally and developed multiple pulmonary metastatic tumors.[92,94] Therefore, the immune response evoked against H-2D^b antigens failed to reject the locally growing tumor mass, but was efficient to control the growth of the metastatic tumor cells. It is of interest that following i.v. inoculation of 3LL tumor cells into naive allogeneic mice experimental pulmonary metastases developed equally regardless of the H-2 haplotype of the recipients. However, when 3LL cells were inoculated i.v. into allogenic mice after resection of the local 3LL tumor, the formation of experimetnal metastases in the lungs was completely prevented.[93]

Analysis of H-2^b antigen expression by tumor cells derived from the individual metastatic foci which developed in the syngeneic C57BL/6 mice revealed that some metastatic foci contained tumor cells with high H-2^b antigens whereas others had low expression. The metastatic ability of these tumor cells was assessed by intrafootpad inoculation into syngeneic mice followed by excision of local 8 to 10 mm tumor. M-3LL with high H-2^b antigen expression grew faster locally and developed more postoperative tumor metastases that L-3LL or M-3LL with low H-2^b antigen expression.[40] Similar results were obtained when local and metastatic growth of L-3LL tumor cells sorted by FACS-II was tested. The sorted fraction of L-3LL with high H-2^b antigen expression had a higher rate of local and metastatic growth than the L-3LL cells with low expression of MHC products.[40]

These results were obtained without discrimination of the relative expression of H-2K^b and H-2D^b gene products. When metastatic ability and expression of both ends of H-2 complex were analyzed using numerous clones and subclones of 3LL tumor, the data demonstrated that the metastatic potential of selected clone populations did not depend entirely on the absolute levels of class I H-2^b antigens, but rather correlated with the level of imbalance in expression of H-2K^b and H-2D^b gene products.[95] High metastatic clones expressed relatively low levels of H-2K^b antigens and relatively high level of H-2D^b. However, three clones had low H-2K^b expression, but were nonmetastatic. It was found that these clones had also low level of H-2D^b antigens. Therefore, based on this study it was concluded that a "low K^b/high D^b" phenotype is highly metastatic, whereas a low K^b/low D^b" and "high K^b/high D^b" phenotypes are nonmetastatic. Intermediate metastatic ability was associated with medium K^b/high D^b antigen expression.[95]

The relevance of these associations between H-2 antigen expression and metastatic ability of tumor cells can also be expressed on the basis of their immunogenicity. In this connection, the immunogenicity of low and high metastatic clones was compared.[96] Clone A9, selected from 3LL tumor, expressed both H-2K^b and H-2D^b antigens was found to be immunogenic and nonmetastatic, whereas clone D122 expressed only H-2D^b antigens and was nonimmunogenic and highly metastatic.[96]

The association between MHC gene product expression and metastatic ability was clearly demonstrated with another experimental tumor, T-10 sarcoma, induced by methylcholanthrene in a (C57BL/6J × C3HeB/FeJ) F1 mouse.[97-99] It is expected that this tumor should express both parental H-2 haplotypes, namely H-2^b/H-2^k antigens. Comparison of H-2 antigen expression by locally growing T-10 tumor cells (L-T10) and tumor cells derived from pulmonary metastases (M-T10) showed that L-T10 tumor cells expressed only H-2^b but not H-2^k antigens, whereas M-T10 had both H-2^b/H-2^k antigens.[97,98] Further studies demonstrated that L-T10 tumor cells lack both H-2K^k and H-2D^k molecules. In contrast, M-T10 expressed H-2K^k and H-2D^k products.[97,98] The acquisition of H-2^k antigens by metastatic cells could be a result of re-expression of H-2^k genes during metastatic spread and growth or of pre-existence of these metastatic cells within the primary L-T10 tumor cell population.

Studies of clones of the L-T10 tumor revealed that eight out of ten selected clones were H-2^b positive, but H-2^k negative. Two clones were found to express both H-2^b and H-2^k haplotypes.[97,98] Only clones which expressed both haplotypes were found to be metastatic. The nonmetastatic phenotype of H-2^k negative clones appeared to be due not to their inability to proliferate in the lungs but rather their sensitivity to immune destruction. Indeed, the H-2^b positive but H-2^k negative clones were able to develop multiple metastases in immunosuppressed irradiated (450R) mice. Metastatic cells derived from immunosuppressed mice were also H-2^k negative.[98]

Detailed analysis of expression of K- and D-ends of both H-2^b/H-2^k haplotypes among the selected clones indicate that metastatic H-2^b/H-2^k positive clones express only H-2D^b/H-2D^k antigens, whereas K^k and K^b end molecules of these haplotypes were missing. Nonmetastatic clones as well as original L-T10 tumor cells which are H-2^b positive and H-2^k negative also did not express H-2K^b genes in addition to their lack of H-2K^k and H-2D^k products.[99]

When the stability of these properties was investigated, the following results were obtained: metastatic clones retained their metastatic properties and their profile of H-2 antigen expression for 15 to 25 serial passages in syngeneic F1 mice. However, upon further transplantation, H-2^k negative clones shifted to expression of the H-2^k haplotype and in parallel acquired the capacity to produce pulmonary metastases.[99]

The differences in H-2 antigen expression and metastatic behavior were closely associated with the immunogenic properties of the investigated clones. T10 clones which expressed H-2D^b antigen were immunogenic and nonmetastatic, whereas clones with H-2D^b and H-2D^k antigens were nonimmunogenic and highly metastatic.[119]

All these experiments indicate that the expression of some H-2 gene products on the cell surface of tumor cells influences their immunogenicity and metastatic behavior. More direct evidence of the relationship between these parameters came from the experiments with H-2 gene transfection into T-10 tumor cells.[100] Since metastatic and nonmetastatic clones did not express K^b and K^k antigens, the effect of H-2K^b and H-2K^k gene transfer on the tumorigenic, metastatic, and immunogenic properties of these clones was investigated. As a result, the transfected clones expressed K-end gene products and the metastatic clone lost its ability to form pulmonary metastases in the immunocompetent mice, but not in the immunosuppressed irradiated (550R) syngeneic mice. Suppression of metastatic behavior was observed following transfection with either K^k or K^b genes.[100] Expression of K-end gene products in the metastatic and nonmetastatic clone increased their immunogenicity and decreased their tumorigenic properties. However, reduction in tumorigenicity was found mostly when clones were transfected with H-2K^b and less with H-2K^k gene. Clones transfected with K^b or K^k were able to immunize and induce resistance to subsequent challenge. Specific CTL were derived from spleen cells of immune mice. These CTL were cytotoxic only for transfected metastatic and nonmetastatic clones, whereas no effect was found when H-2K negative clones or H-2K positive but nonrelated tumor cells were used as a targets. The sensitivity to CTL of transfected metastatic and nonmetastatic clones expressing K-end antigens suggests that these clones shared TATA.[100] Thus, the appearance of K-end antigens converted metastatic tumor cells into nonmetastatic cells. In contrast, the presence of D^k antigens had the opposite effect and was observed only in the metastatic clones. The different effect of K- and D-end genes on the metastatic properties of tumor cells may be attributable to the different physiological functions of these molecules with mostly immunogenic activity of the K-end product and suppressogenic activity of the D^k products.[97-99,100,118]

During the last 20 years, the B16 melanoma served as one of the most useful experimental systems to study the mechanisms involved in the metastatic process. Selection of the sublines of B16 melanoma with high and low metastatic ability stimulated numerous investigations to understand the mechanisms responsible for the differences in metastatic characteristics among these sublines. The highly metastatic subline, B16F10, was selected following ten consequantive i.v. transfers of metastatic cells derived from the lungs of inoculated mice.[101] If MHC antigens play a role in the determination of the metastatic phenotype, it would be expected that low and high metastatic sublines of B16 melanoma would differ in their expression of MHC gene products.

Table 1
H-2 ANTIGEN EXPRESSION ON THE CELL SURFACE
OF B16 MELANOMA CELL VARIANTS

		% Positive cells	
Tumor	Characterisitics	H-2K^b	H-2D^b
B16	Initial low metastatic population	31.6[a]	26.9
B16F1	Low metastatic subline	20.6	24.5
B16F10	Selected on high lung colonization	3.5	9.1
B16F10^{Lr}	Selected by resistance to lymphocyte-mediated cytotoxicity	9.8	11.9
BL6	Selected from B16F10 by high invasiveness	1.2	10.1
BL6T2	BL6 treated with MNNG	47.4	76.5
BL6inf	BL6 treated with interferon	53.9	93.6

[a]   The expression of H-2K^b and H-2D^b antigens on the cell surface of B16 melanoma cell variants was analyzed by use of monoclonal antibodies and flow cytometry.

Baniyash et al.[102] using complement dependent cytotoxicity, radioimmunobinding and quantitative absorbtion assays have found that low metastatic B16F1 melanoma cells had higher levels of H-2^b antigen expression than high metastatic B16F10 melanoma cells.

Using monoclonal antibodies and flow cytometry analysis, we investigated H-2^b antigen expression by various B16 melanoma sublines (Table 1). The results of this study indicated that the original B16 melanoma and the B16F1 subline had higher levels of H-2K^b and H-2D^b antigens than did B16F10 and BL6 melanoma sublines selected for high metastatic and invasive properties. After in vivo treatment of BL6 melanoma cells with N-methyl-N'-nitro-nitrosoguanidine (MNNG), the expression of class I antigens of H-2^b complex dramatically increased. In parallel, MNNG-treated BL6 melanoma cells (BL6T2) became poorly metastatic.[103,104]

High levels of H-2^b anitgen expression and the low metastatic ability of BL6T2 melanoma cells was associated with their high immunogenicity. After inoculation of 1 × 10^5 BL6T2 melanoma cells, tumors were rejected in 70% of C57BL/6 recipients.[103] With an increase of the dose of inoculation (5 × 10^5 cells), progressively growing tumors developed in 60% of C57BL/6 mice. After removal of local BL6T2 tumors, almost all of the operated C57BL/6 mice remained free from metastases. Suppression of NK reactivity in these mice by treatment with anti-asialo GM-1 serum did not effect metastasis formation, since the metastatic cells were already eliminated by T-cells.

The involvement of T-cell-mediated immunity in the control of BL6T2 metastatic spread and growth was suppported by the observation that BL6T2 melanoma cells were able to grow and metastasize in 100% of nude mice. However, in the absence of T-lymphocytes NK cells appeared to be responsible for antimetastatic defense, since after anti-asailo GM-1 treatment, the number of metastatic foci in the lungs of nude mice further increased. In the absence of T-cell immunity and suppression of NK reactivity of nude mice, no difference in the metastatic potentials between BL6 and BL6T2 melanoma cells was observed.

Treatment of BL6 melanoma cells with interferon also induced high levels of class I H-2^b antigen expression (Table 1), but did not influence their immunogenic and metastatic properties. This discrepancy can be explained by the fact that effect of interferon on H-2 antigen expression was transient and the level of H-2K^b products returned to the initial low levels by 7 days after interferon withdrawal.[122]

Although, for some tumor cell sublines, a positive correlation between the level of MHC antigen expression and metastatic ability could be found, it is necessary to keep in mind that the level of MHC products could be just one among many properties which determine the metastatic potential of tumor cells. Indeed, B16F10^{Lr} melanoma cells was selected from the highly metastatic B16F10 subline on the basis of resistance to lysis by immune lymphocytes[105] maintained low levels of H-2^b antigen expression, but they gained or lost other properties which converted them into low metastatic cells (Table 1).

The analysis of MHC antigen expression by human malignant cells also demonstrated the substantial heterogeneity in the expression of MHC antigen among tumor cells derived from the primary and metastatic lesions.[79,80,83]

Parmiani et al.[83] found that human melanoma cells derived from the primary and metastatic tumors expressed high levels of MHC class I products, but they showed significant variability in the expression of class II HLA-DR and melanoma associated antigens.

The HLA-DR molecules on the primary and metastatic melanoma cells had different physiological functions. Only DR-poisitive primary tumor cells were able to stimulate the autologous lymphocytes to proliferate. In addition, stimulated lymphocytes became specifically cytotoxic against autologous melanoma cells. In contrast, neither DR-positive nor DR-negative metastatic cells were able to stimulate autologous PBL. Moreover, DR-positive metastatic cells suppressed the proliferation of PBL stimulated by allogeneic cells or interlukin-2 (IL-2).[83] Thus, tumor cells which provide suppressogenic rather than immunogenic stimuli might have some advantages during the metastatic migration and growth.

B. MHC Antigens and Recognition of "Self", "Nonself", and "No Self" in Association with Metastatic Process

The functional importance of MHC antigens on the cell surface is mostly associated with "self" identification of somatic cells in the multicellular organism by controlling the recognition of cell membrane components of normal or malignant cells by T-cell-mediated immunity.

MHC antigens can guide the specific immune lymphocyte for recognition of foreign antigens and elimination of "nonself" cells.[76] Therefore, MHC loss variants of tumor cells are not recognizable by the T-cell immune system, and thus could escape immune destruction. Similary, virus-infected cells missing MHC-restricted elements are less likely to be eliminated by the host. Cells which partially or completely lost their MHC antigens may be termed as "no self" cells.[113] These cells could be eliminated by mechanisms independent of the T-cell system. It is considered that NK cells and macrophages can destroy malignant or virus infected cells in a MHC nonrestricted manner.[106] Numerous experimental data indicate that NK cells could represent the effective mechanism which can restrict the survival and propagation of normal or malignant cells lacking all or some elements of MHC system.

Many experiments have been performed in which F1 hybrid mice were inoculated with parental cells that express only one of the H-2 haplotypes expressed by F1 hybrid host. Higher resistance of semisyngeneic F1 mice against parental tumor grafts in comparison to syngeneic host was first demonstrated by Snell and Stevens.[107] Later, it was found that F1 hybrids are able to reject parental normal bone marrow cells.[108] Similarly, survival of leukemia cells was lower when they were inoculated into F1 hybrid mice than into the syngeneic parental recipients.[109][111] The hybrid resistance to normal bone marrow cells was shown to be due to recognition of Hh antigens controlled by H-2D-linked recessive genes.[108] The rejection of semisyngeneic normal or malignant cells of F1 recipients was found to mediated not by T-cell immunity but mostly by NK cells.[109-112]

Elimination of semisyngeneic grafts in F1 hosts was substantially reduced in beige mice and in mice where NK reactivity was depressed by pretreatment with anti-asialo GM-1 serum.[112]

Based on this finding Kärre et al.[113] hypothesized that the hybrid resistance phenomenon reflected an in vivo mechanism in which NK cells destroyed normal cells which were unable to present in full the MHC antigens of the host.

Similarly, H-2 negative tumor cells could also be recognized as the "absence of self" and thereby be a prime subject of attack by NK cells whereas T-lymphocytes would be unable to destroy such tumor cells.[113] This hypothesis includes an additional assumption that MHC products can diminish or switch off susceptibility to the cytotoxic effects of NK cells.[113] Based on this suggestion, H-2 negative normal or malignant cells were postulated should have higher levels of susceptibility to the cytotoxic action of NK cells then H-2 positive cells. Several experimental data support this hypothesis. Cortical thymocytes which have low H-2 antigen expression are more sensitive than H-2 high medullary thymocytes to the cytotoxic activity of NK cells.[114] H-2 negative teratocarcinoma cells can be destroyed by NK cells, but their susceptibility reduced with the appearance of H-2 antigens.[115]

In order to further confirm these observations, Ljunggren and Kärre[116] selected H-2 negative variants of EL4 and RBL-5 lymphomas after mutagenesis with ethylmethane methane sulfonate (EMS) and exposure to anti-H-2 antibodies and complement. These variants were rather stable under in vitro or in vivo conditions. Although H-2 positive and H-2 negative variants of EL4 or RBL-5 lymphomas had similar growth characteristics in vitro, H-2 negative variants in contrast to H-2 positive variants failed to grow in the syngeneic mice after inoculation of $1 \times 10^3 - 1 \times 10^5$ cells. It required inoculation of 10^6 cells to produce progressively growing tumors. It seems that non-T-cell-mediated immunity is responsible for this rejection. First of all, H-2 negative variants were nonimmunogenic, in contrast to H-2 positive cells which were able to induce specific immune resistance. Secondly, rejection of H-2 negative cells of EL4 and RBL-5 lymphomas cells ($10^4 - 10^6$) was also observed in nude mice. However, growth of these H-2 negative variants was found in nude mice whose NK reactivity was depressed by pretreatment with anti-asialo GM-1 serum. Additional test for the NK-mediated intravascular elimination of tumor cells indicate that after i.v. inoculation, survival of radiolabeled H-2 negative tumor cells in different organs was 5- to 100-fold lower than H-2 positive cells. The differences in survival disappeared when these cells were inoculated into mice pretreated with anti-asialo GM-1 serum.[116]

An inverse correlation between H-2 antigen expression and NK sensitivity of tumor cells was also found when these parameters were investigated with YAC-1 lymphoma cells. YAC-1 cells maintains high levels of sensitivity to NK cells in parallel with low levels of H-2^a antigen expression during in vitro cultivation. After a single in vivo passage YAC-1 cells increased the level of H-2^a antigens and became resistant to NK-mediated cytotoxicity. Explantation of YAC ascites into tissue culture was associated with a decrease in H-2^a antigen expression and an increase in their NK sensitivity.[117]

Using mutagenic EMS treatment and selection with anti-H-2^a antibodies and complement, two H-2 negative variants of YAC lymphoma cells were obtained.[118] These variants and low H-2^a parental YAC-1 cells were similar in their sensitivity to NK cells. However, parental YAC-1 cells, after interferon treatment or in vivo passage, increased the H-2 antigen expression and became NK resistant, whereas H-2^a negative variants under interferon treatment or in vivo passage did not increase either H-2^a expression nor resistance to NK-mediated killing.[118]

Similar observations were made when B16 melanoma cells were investigated. B16 melanoma cells derived from in vivo growing tumor expressed relatively high levels of H-2 antigens and resistance to NK activity. During in vitro culture, the level of H-2 antigen expression declined with parallel increase in sensitivity to NK cells.[120] These changes were also associated with the alteration of their metastatic ability. High H-2^b B16 melanoma cells produced more metastases in the lungs than NK-sensitive H-2^b low B16 melanoma cells. Treatment of B16 melanoma cells with interferon increased H-2^b antigen expression, decreased their NK sensitivity and increased their metastatic ability.[120]

Sensitivity of tumor cells to the cytotoxic action of NK cells probably depends on several properties of the tumor cell membrane. As an example, it was demonstrated that although some YAC-1 cell variants had low level of H-2 antigens, they were resistant to NK cells. This resistance was associated with relatively high levels of sialic acid on the cell membrane of these variants.[121]

In our experiments, B16 melanoma cells treated with MNNG had high levels of H-2^b antigens but was more sensitive to NK cells and less metastatic than H-2 negative parental B16 melanoma. This NK resistance of H-2 negative B16 melanoma was associated with higher levels of sialic acid on their cell membrane.[122] Although B16F1 and B16F10 cells differ in their H-2 antigen expression and metastatic potential,[104] these tumor sublines did not show significant differences in NK sensitivity.[44,45]

Nevertheless, the inverse correlation between the H-2 antigen expression and NK sensitivity of some tumor cells could shed light on some previously unexplainable associations between MHC antigen expression and metastatic ability of tumor cells.

In order to understand the divergent data concerning MHC antigen expression on metastatic tumor cells, it is necessary to take into consideration that both specific T-cell and nonspecific natural mediated immunity could be involved in the selection of the metastatic cell population. In addition, high levels of MHC antigen expression by tumor cells does not necessarily indicate that they have high immunogenic properties. Immunogenicity of tumor cells depends not only upon the level of expression of MHC restricted elements but also upon the level of expression of TATA. Immunoselection mediated by T-lymphocytes during metastasis formation could be directed against both MHC and TATA. Therefore, the expected low expression of MHC antigens by metastatic cells as a result of immunoselection is not always observed.

Immunogenic tumor cells can develop metastases as a result of selection of tumor cells

1.   With low levels of MHC, but high TATA expression
2.   With high levels of MHC but low levels of TATA
3.   With high levels of MHC and with TATA different from the primary tumor specificity
4.   With low levels of both MHC and TATA expression

NK cells also can participate in the formation of the population of metastatic cells by elimination of relatively sensitive tumor cells. Preferential negative selection of tumor cells with "absence of self" will result in appearance of metastases which expressed higher levels of MHC gene products than primary tumor cells did. Indeed, locally growing T-10 tumor of F1 origin expressed only H-2^b and missing H-2^k haplotype, whereas metastases from this tumor had H-2^b/H-2^k antigens.[97-100] Comparison of the metastatic ability and H-2 antigen expression among the individual clones from T-10 tumor again demonstrated that cells with absence of one of the parental haplotypes were unable to develop pulmonary metastases.

Although in vitro all T-10 clones were resistant to the cytotoxic action of normal spleen cells, the results of investigation of the rate of tumor cell elimination fit this prediction. Clone IB9, which express both H-2D^b and H-2D^k antigens was metastatic and the number of these radiolabeled tumor cells which survived in the lungs 4 hr after their inoculation was three to four times higher than the number of cells of clone IC9 and IID6, which express only 2-D^b antigens.[99] It is of interest that after 36 in vitro passage, clones IC9 and IID6 became H-2D^b and H-2D^k positive, and this was associated with an increase in the survival of these tumor cells in the lungs and the development of metastatic foci in the lungs.[99] Involvement of NK cells in the control of metastasis formation by T-10 clones was supported by the finding that stimulation of NK reactivity by poly I:C inhibited the metastatic growth whereas suppression of NK cell function by cyclophosphamide caused a substantial increase in the formation of pulmonary metastases by metastatic and nonmetastatic T-10 clones.[119] The inverse correlation between immunogenicity of the T-10 clones and their metastatic properties indicates that specific T-cell-mediated immunity also was involved in the formation of the phenotype of metastatic tumor cell population.[99,100,119]

Thus, MHC gene products might play a role in realization of metastatic potential of tumor cells. Both the specific T-cell-mediated and natural immunity could be involved in the control of metastatic spread and growth. The possible interaction of these two effector mechanisms in the selection of metastatic cell population need to be considered in order to understand the results pertaining to investigation of the role of the MHC gene products in metastatic behavior of tumor cells.

REFERENCES

1. Weiss, L., Metastatic inefficiency, in: *Cancer Invasion and Metastasis,* Liotta, L. and Hart, I., Eds., Martines Nijhoff Publishers, Hingham, Mass., 1982, 81.
2. Salsbury, A., The significance of the circulating cancer cell, *Cancer Treat. Rev.,* 2, 55, 1975.
3. Fidler, I., Metastasis: quantitive analysis of distribution and fate of tumor emboli labeled with ^{125}I-S-iodo-2'deoxyuridine, *J. Natl. Cancer Inst.,* 45, 773, 1970.
4. Fidler, I., Gerstein, D., and Hart, I., The biology of cancer invasion and metastasis, *Adv. Cancer Res.,* 28, 149, 1978.
5. Liotta, L., Thorgeirsson, U., and Garbisa, S., Role of collagenases in tumor cell invasion, *Cancer Met. Rev.,* 1, 277, 1982.
6. Nicolson, G., Cancer metastasis: organ colonization and cell-surface properties of malignant cells, *Biochim. Biophys. Acta,* 695, 113, 1982.
7. Schirrmacher, V., Cancer metastasis: experimetnal approaches, theoretical concepts and impacts for treatment strategies, *Adv. Cancer Res.,* 43, 1, 1985.
8. Eccles, S. and Alexander, P., Immunologically mediated restraint of latent tumor metastasis, *Nature (London),* 257, 52, 1975.
9. Kim, U., Baumler, A., Carruthers, C., and Bielat, K., Immunological escape mechanism in spontaneously metastasizing mammary tumors, *Proc. Natl. Acad. Sci. U.S.A.,* 72, 1012, 1975.
10. Fidler, I. and Kripke, M., Tumor cell antigenicity, host immunity and cancer metastasis, *Cancer Immunol. Immunother.,* 7, 201, 1980.
11. Schirrmacher, V., Fogel, M., Russman, E., Boslet, K., Altevogt, P., and Beck, L., Antigenic variation in cancer metastasis: immune escape versus immune control, *Cancer Met. Rev.,* 1, 241, 1982.
12. Fidler, I., Gersten, D., and Kripke, M., Influence of immune status on the metastasis of three murine fibrosarcomas of different immunogenicities, *Cancer Res.,* 39, 3816, 1979.
13. Ford, C. and Hamerton, J., Colchicine, hypotonic citrate, squash sequence for mammalian chromosomes, *Stain Technol.,* 31, 247, 1956.
14. Levan, A., Chromosomes in cancer tissue, *Ann. N.Y. Acad. Sci.,* 63, 774, 1956.
15. Makino, S., The concept of stemline cells as progenitors of a neoplastic population, in *Cytologia,* Proc. Internat. Genet. Symp. Tokyo, 1956, 177.
16. Hauschka, T., The chromosome in ontogeny and oncogeny, *Cancer Res.,* 21, 957, 1961.
17. Nowell, P., The clonal evolution of tumor cell populations, *Science,* 194, 23, 1976.

18. Cifone, M. and Fidler, I., Increasing metastatic potential is associated with increasing genetic instability of clones isolated from murine neoplasms, *Proc. Natl. Acad. Sci. U.S.A.,* 78, 6949, 1981.

19. Ling, V., Chambers, A., Harris, J., and Hill, R., Quantitative genetic analysis of tumor progression, *Cancer Met. Rev.,* 4, 173, 1985.

20. Poste, G. and Greig, R., On the genesis and regulation of cellular heterogeneity in malignant tumors, *Invasion Met.,* 2, 137, 1982.

21. Heppner, G., Tumor heterogeneity, *Cancer Res.,* 44, 2259, 1984.

22. Kerbel, R., Implications of immunological heterogeneity of tumours, *Nature (London),* 280, 358, 1979.

23. Frost, P. and Kerbel, R., On the possible epigenetic mechanism(s) of tumor cell heterogeneity, *Cancer Met. Rev.,* 2, 375, 1984.

24. Hauschka, T. and Levan, A., Inverse relationship between chromosome ploidy and host-specificity of sixteen transplantable tumors, *Exp. Cell Res.,* 4, 457, 1953.

25. Klein, G. and Klein, E., Histocompatibility changes in tumors, *J. Cell. Comp. Physiol.,* 52, 125, 1958.

26. Prehn, R., Analysis of antigenic heterogeneity with individual 3-methylcholanthrene-induced mouse sarcoma, *J. Natl. Cancer Inst.,* 45, 1039, 1970.

27. Miller, F., Intratumor heterogeneity, *Cancer Met. Rev.,* 1, 319, 1982.

28. Lobko, G., Alteration of the genetic structure of tumor cell populations by lymphoid cells of tumor bearing mice, in *Proc. Med. Genet. Human Genet.,* Rockitsky, P., Ed., Science and Technik, Minsk, 1971, 276.

29. Gorelik, L., Study the genetic mechanisms of susceptibility (resistance) of tumor cell populations to the humoral antibodies of tumor-bearing mice, in *Proc. Med. Genet. Human Genet.,* Rockitsky, P., Ed., Science and Technik, Minsk, 1971, 221.

30. Olsson, L. and Ebbesen, P., Natural polyclonality of spontaneous AKR leukemia and its consequences for so-called specific immunotherapy, *J. Natl. Cancer Inst.,* 62, 623, 1979.

31. Pimm, M. and Baldwin, R., Antigenic differences between primary methycholanthrene-induced rat sarcomas and post-surgical recurrences, *Int. J. Cancer,* 20, 37, 1977.

32. Dennis, J., Donaghue, T., and Kerbel, R., An examination of tumor antigen loss in spontaneous metastasis, *Invasion Met.,* 2, 111, 1981.

33. Deichman, G. and Kluchareva, T., Loss of transplantation antigen in primary simian virus 40-induced tumors and their metastases, *J. Natl. Cancer Inst.,* 36, 647, 1966.

34. Albino, A., Lloyd, K., Houghton, A., Oettgen, H., and Old, L., Heterogeneity in surface antigen and glycoprotein expression of cell lines derived from different melanoma metastases of the same patient. Implications for the study of tumor antigen, *J. Exp. Med.,* 154, 1764, 1981.

35. Primus, K., Kuhns, W., and Goldenberg, D., Immunological heterogeneity of carcinoembryonic antigen: immunohistochemical detection of carcinoembryonic antigen determinants in colonic tumors with monoclonal antibodies, *Cancer Res.,* 43, 693, 1983.

36. Roth, J., Restrepo, C., Scuderi, P., Baldwin, R., Reichert, C., and Hosoi, S., Analysis of antigenic expression by primary and autologous metastasis human sarcomas using murine monoclonal antibodies, *Cancer Res.,* 44, 5320, 1984.

37. Sugarbaker, E. and Cohen, A., Altered antigenicity in spontaneous pulmonary metastases from an antigenic murine sarcoma, *Surgery,* 72, 155, 1972.

38. Fogel, M., Gorelik, E., Segal, S., and Feldman, M., Cell-surface antigens of tumor metastasis differ from those of the local tumor, *J. Natl. Cancer Inst.,* 62, 385, 1979.

39. Gorelik, E., Fogel, M., DeBaetselier, P., Katzav, S., Feldman, M., and Segal, S., Immunobiological diversity of metastatic cells, in *Cancer Invasion and Metastasis,* Liotte, L. and Hart, I., Eds., Martinus Nijhoff, Hingham, Mass., 1982, 134.

40. Pimm, M., Embleton, M., and Baldwin, R., Multiple antigenic specificities within primary 3-methylcholanthrene-induced rat sarcomas and metastases, *Int. J. Cancer,* 25, 621, 1981.

41. Gorelik, E., Concomitant tumor immunity and the resistance to a second tumor challenge, *Adv. Cancer Res.,* 39, 71, 1983.

42. North, R. and Bursuker, I., Generation and decay of the immune response to a progressive fibrosarcoma. I. Ly 1⁺2⁻ suppressor T-cells down regulate the generation of Ly1⁻2⁺ effector T cells, *J. Exp. Med.,* 159, 1295, 1984.

43. Gorelik, E., Wiltrout, R., Okumura, K., Habu, S., and Herberman, R., Role of NK cells in the control of metastatic spread and growth of tumor cells in mice, *Int. J. Cancer,* 30, 107, 1982.

44. Hanna, N. and Fidler, I., The role of natural killer cells in the destruction of circulating tumor emboli, *J. Natl. Cancer Inst.,* 65, 801, 1980.

45. Hanna, N., Role of natural killer cells in control of cancer metastasis, *Cancer Met. Rev.,* 1, 45, 1982.

46. Riccardi, C., Pucceti, P., Santoni, A., and Herberman, R., Rapid *in vivo* assay of mouse NK cell activity, *J. Natl. Cancer Inst.,* 63, 1041, 1979.

47. Gorelik, E. and Herberman, R., Role of Natural Killer (NK) cells in the control of tumor growth and metastatic spread, in *Basic and Clinical Immunology,* Vol. 2, Herberman, R., Ed., Martinus Nijhoff, Hingham, Mass., in press.

48. Brown, J. and Parker, E., Host treatments affecting artificial pulmonary metastases: interpretation of loss of radioactively labelled cells from lungs, *Br. J. Cancer,* 40, 677, 1979.

49. Pollack, S., Direct evidence for anti-tumor acitvity by NK cells *in vivo*: growth of B16 melanoma in anti-NK 1.1 treated mice, in *NK Cell and Other Natural Effector Cells,* Herberman, R., Ed., Academic Press, New York, 1982, 1347.

50. Gorelik, E., Bere, E., and Herberman, R., Role of NK cells in the antimetastatic effect of anticoagulant drugs, *Int. J. Cancer,* 33, 87, 1982.

51. Talmadge, J. E., Meyers, K. M., Prieur, D. J., and Starkey, J. R., Role of NK cells in tumour growth and metastasis in beige mice, *Nature (London),* 284, 622, 1980.

52. Djeu, J. Y., Heinbaugh, J. A., Holden, H. T., and Herberman, R. B., Role of macrophages in the augmentation of mouse natural killer cell activity by poly I:C and interferon, *J. Immunol.,* 122, 182, 1979.

53. Hanna, H. and Burton, R., Definitive evidence that natural killer (NK) cells inhibit experimental tumor metastasis *in vivo, J. Immunol.,* 127, 1754, 1981.

54. Barlozzari, T., Reynolds, C., and Herberman, R., *In vivo,* role of natural killer cells: involvement of large granular lymphocytes in the clearance of tumor cells in anti-asialo GM_1-treated rats, *J. Immunol.,* 131, 1024, 1983.

55. Chow, D., Brown, G., and Greenberg, A., NK cell and NAB antitumor activity *in vivo,* in *NK Cells and Other Natural Effector Cells,* Herberman, R., Ed., Academic Press, New York, 1982, 1379.

56. Korec, S., The role of granulocytes in host defense against tumors, in *Natural Cell-Mediated Immunity Against Tumors,* Herberman, R., Ed., Academic Press, New York, 1980, 1301.

57. Gorelik, E., Fogel, M., Feldman, M., and Segal, S., Differences in resistance of metastatic tumor cells and cells from local tumor growth to cytotoxicity of natural killer cells, *J. Natl. Cancer Inst.,* 63, 1397, 1979.

58. Brodt, P., Feldman, M., and Segal, S., Differences in the metastatic potential of two sublines of tumor 3LL selected for resistance to natural NK-like effector cells, *Cancer Immunol. Immunother.,* 16, 109, 1983.

59. Gorelik, E., Feldman, M., and Segal, S., Selection of 3LL tumor subline resistant to natural effector cells concomitantly selected for increased metastatic potency, *Cancer Immunol. Immunother.,* 12, 105, 1982.

60. Brooks, C., Flannery, G., Wilmott, N., Austin, E., Kenwrick, S., and Baldwin, R., Tumour cells in metastatic deposits with altered sensitivity to natural killer cells, *Int. J. Cancer,* 28, 191, 1981.

61. Teale, D., Rees, R., Clark, A., Walker, J., and Potter, C., Reduced susceptibility to natural killer cell lysis of hamster tumours exhibiting high levels of spontaneous metastasis, *Cancer Lett.,* 19, 221, 1983.

62. Hanna, N. and Fidler, I., Relationship between metastatic potential and resistance to natural killer cell-mediated cytotoxicity in three murine tumor systems, *J. Natl. Cancer Inst.,* 66, 1183, 1981.

63. Segal, S., Kingsmore, S., Gorelik, E., and Feldman, M., Control by NK cells of the generation of lung metastases by the Lewis lung carcinoma, in *Current Concepts in Human Immunology and Cancer Immunomodulation,* Serrou, B., Ed., Elsevier/North Holland, Amsterdam, 1982, 227.

64. Alexander, P., The functions of the macrophage in malignant disease, *Ann. Rev. Med.,* 27, 207, 1976.

65. Miner, K., Klostergaard, J., Granger, G., and Nicolson, G., Differences in cytotoxic effects of activated murine peritoneal macrophages and J774 monocyte cells on metastatic variants of B16 melanoma, *J. Natl. Cancer Inst.,* 68, 507, 1983.

66. Miner, K. and Nicolson, G., Differences in the sensitivities of murine metastatic lymphoma/lymphosarcoma variants to macrophage mediated cytolysis and/or cytostasis, *Cancer Res.,* 43, 2063, 1983.

67. Yamamura, Y., Fisher, B., Harnaha, J., and Proctor, J., Heterogeneity of murine mammary adenocarcinoma cell subpopulations. *In vitro* and *in vivo* resistance to macrophage cytotoxicity and its association with metastatic capacity, *Int. J. Cancer,* 33, 67, 1984.

68. Montovani, A., *In vitro* effects on tumor cells of macrophages isolated from an early passage chemically induced murine sarcoma and from its spontaneous metastases, *Int. J. Cancer,* 27, 221, 1981.

69. Hibbs, J., Charman, H., and Weinberg, J., The macrophage as an antineoplastic surveillance cell: biological perspectives, *J. Reticoloendothel. Soc.,* 24, 549, 1978.

70. Fidler, I., Therapy of spontaneous metastases by intravenous injection of liposomes containing lymphokines, *Science,* 208, 1469, 1980.

71. Urban, J. and Schreiber, H., Selection of macrophage-resistant progressor tumor variants by the normal host, *J. Exp. Med.,* 157, 642, 1983.

72. Wiltrout, R., Brunda, M., and Holden, H., Variation in selectivity of tumor cell cytolysis by murine macrophages, macrophage-like cell lines, and NK cells, *Int. J. Cancer*, 30, 335, 1982.
73. Reading, C., Brunson, K., Torriani, M., and Nicolson, G., Malignancies of metastatic murine lymphosarcoma cell lines and clones correlate with decreased cell surface display of RNA tumor virus envelope glycoprotein gp70, *Proc. Natl. Acad. Sci. U.S.A.*, 77, 5943, 1980.
74. Reading, C., Kraemer, P., Miner, K., and Nicolson, G., *In vivo* and *in vitro* properties of malignant variants of RAW117 metastatic murine lymphoma/lymphosarcoma, *Clin. Exp. Met.*, 1, 135, 1983.
75. North, S. and Nicolson, G., Heterogeneity in the sensitivities of the 13762NF rat mammary adenocarcinoma cell clones to cytolysis mediated by extra- and intratumor macrophages, *Cancer Res.*, 45, 1453, 1985.
76. Doherty, P., Knowles, B., and Wettstein, P., Immunological surveillance of tumors in the context of major histocompatibility complex restriction of T cell function, *Adv. Cancer Res.*, 42, 1, 1984.
77. Festenstein, H. and Schmidt, W., Variation of MHC antigenic profiles of tumor cells and its biological effects, *Immunol. Rev.*, 60, 85, 1981.
78. Martin, W., Structural and functional alterations in H-2 antigen expression on tumor cells, *Transplant. Proc.*, 15, 2097, 1983.
79. Natali, P., Bigotti, A., Nicorta, M., Viora, M., Manfredi, D., and Ferrone, S., Distribution of human class I (HLA-A, B, C) histocompatibility antigens in normal and malignant tissues of nonlymphoid origin, *Cancer Res.*, 44, 4679, 1984.
80. Lampson, L., Fisher, C., and Whelan, J., Striking paucity of HLA-A,B,C and β_2-microglobulin on human neuroblastoma cell lines, *J. Immunol.*, 130, 2471, 1983.
81. Sanderson, A. and Beverly, P., Interferon, β_2-microglobulin and immunoselection in the pathway to malignancy, *Immunol. Today*, 8, 211, 1983.
82. Doyle, A., Martin, J., Fune, K., Gazdat, A., Carney, D., Martin, S., Linnoila, I., Cuttitta, F., Mulshine, J., Bunn, P., and Minna, J., Markedly decreased expression of class I histocompatibility antigens, protein and mRNA in human small-cell lung cancer, *J. Exp. Med.*, 161, 1135, 1985.
83. Parmiani, G., Fossoti, G., Taramelli, D., Anichini, A., Balsari, A., Gambacorti-Passerini, C., Sciorelli, G., and Cescinelli, N., Autologous cellular immune response to primary and metastatic human melanomas and its regulation by DR antigen expressed on tumor cells, *Cancer Rev.*, 4, 7, 1985.
84. Rogers, M., Gooding, L., Margulies, D., and Evans, G., Analysis of a defect in the H-2 genes of SV40 transformed C3H fibroblasts that do not express H-2K^k, *J. Immunol.*, 130, 2418, 1983.
85. Schrier, P., Bernards, R., Vaessen, R., Houweling, A., and van der Erb, A., Expression of class I major histocompatibility antigens switched off by highly oncogenic adenovirus 12 in transformed rat cells, *Nature (London)*, 305, 771, 1983.
86. Tanaka, K., Isselbacher, K., Khoury, G., and Joy, C., Reversal of oncogenesis by the expression of a major histocompatibility complex class I gene, *Science*, 228, 26, 1985.
87. Hui, K., Grosveld, F., and Festenstein, H., Rejection of transplantable AKR leukemia cells following MHC DNA-mediated transformation, *Nature (London)*, 311, 750, 1984.
88. Axelrad, A. and Klein, G., Differences in histocompatibility requirements between primary tumors and their metastases, *Transplant. Bull.*, 3, 100, 1956.
89. Kraskovsky, G. and Lobko, G., Alteration of the genetic structure of tumor cell population following metastasizing into the regional lymph nodes, in *Genetics of Tumor Growth*, Turbin, N., Rockitsky, P., and Kraskovsky, G., Eds., Science and Technik, Minsk, 1967, 155.
90. Haywood, G. and McKhann, C., Antigenic specificities of murine sarcoma cells. Reciprocal relationship between normal transplantation antigens (H-2) and tumor-specific immunogenicity, *J. Exp. Med.*, 133, 1171, 1971.
91. Gorelik, E., Fogel, M., Segal, S., and Feldman, M., Antigenic differences between local 3LL tumor and its metastases. III. Differences in growth rate in syngeneic, semiallogeneic and allogeneic hosts, 9th Ann. Meet. Israel Immunol. Soc., Tel-Aviv, 35, 38, 1978.
92. Isakov, N., Feldman, M., and Segal, S., Control of progression of local tumor and pulmonary metastasis of the 3LL Lewis lung carcinoma by different histocompatibility requirements in mice, *J. Natl. Cancer Inst.*, 66, 919, 1981.
93. Isakov, N., Katsav, S., Feldman, M., and Segal, S., Loss of expression of transplantation antigens encoded by th H-2K locus on Lewis lung carcinoma cells and its relevance to the tumor's metastatic properties, *J. Natl. Cancer Inst.*, 71, 139, 1983.
94. Isakov, N., Feldman, M., and Segal, S., An immune response against the alloantigens of the 3LL Lewis lung carcinoma prevents the growth of lung metastases but not of local allografts, *Invasion Met.*, 2, 12, 1982.
95. Esenbach, L., Segal, S., and Feldman, M., MHC imbalance and metastatic spread in Lewis lung carcinoma clones, *Int. J. Cancer*, 32, 113, 1983.
96. Eisenbach, L., Hollander, N., Greenfeld, L., Yakor, H., Segal, S., and Feldman, M., The differential expression of H-2K versus H-2D antigens, distinguishing high-metastatic from low-metastatic clones is correlated with the immunogenic properties of the tumor cells, *Int. J. Cancer*, 34, 567, 1984.

97. De Baetselier, P., Katzav, S., Gorelik, E., Feldman, M., and Segal, S., Differential expression of H-2 gene products in tumour cells is associated with their metastogenic properties, *Nature (London),* 288, 179, 1980.

98. Katzav, S., De Baetselier, P., Gorelik, E., Feldman, M., and Segal, S., Immunogenetic control of metastasis formation by a methylcholanthrene-induced tumor (T10) in mice: differential expression of H-2 gene products, *Transplant. Proc.,* 13, 742, 1981.

99. Katzav, S., De Baetselier, P., Tartakovsky, B., Feldman, M., and Segal, S., Alterations in major histocompatibility complex phenotypes of mouse cloned T10 sarcoma cells: association with shifts from nonmetastatic to metastatic cells, *J. Natl. Cancer Inst.,* 71, 317, 1983.

100. Wallich, R., Bulbuc, N., Hämmerling, G., Katzav, S., Segal, S., and Feldman, M., Abrogation of metastatic properties of tumour cells by de novo expression of H-2K antigens following H-2 gene transfection, *Nature (London),* 315, 301, 1985.

101. Fidler, I., Selection of successive tumor lines for metastasis, *Nature (London),* 242, 148, 1973.

102. Raniyash, M., Smorodincky, N., Yankubovioz, M., and Witz, I., Serologically detectable MHC and tumor-associated antigens on B16 melanoma variants and humoral immunity in mice bearing these tumors, *J. Immunol.,* 129, 1318, 1982.

103. Gorelik, E., Peppoloni, S., Overton, R., and Herberman, R., Increase in H-2 antigen expression and immunogenicity of BL6 melanoma cells treated with N-methyl-N'-nitro-nitrosoguanidine, *Cancer Res.,* in press.

104. Gorelik, E., H-2 expression, immunogenicity and metastatic properties of BL6 melanoma cells treated with MNNG, in *Treatment of Metastasis Problems and Prospects,* Hellmann, K., Nicolson, G., and Miles, L., Eds., Taylor and Francis, London, in press.

105. Fidler, I., Gersten, D., and Budmen, M., Characterization in vivo and in vitro of tumor cells selected for resistance to syngeneic lymphocyte-mediated cytotoxicity, *Cancer Res.,* 36, 3160, 1976.

106. Herberman, R., Ed., *NK Cells and Other Natural Effector Cells,* Academic Press, New York, 1982.

107. Snell, G. and Stevens, L., Histocompatibility genes of mice. III. H-1 and H-4 two histocompatibility loci in the first linkage group, *Immunology,* 4, 366, 1961.

108. Cudkowicz, G. and Bennett, M., Peculiar immunobiology of bone marrow allografts. II. Rejection of parental grafts by resistant F1 hybrid mice, *J. Exp. Med.,* 134, 1513, 1971.

109. Carlson, G. and Wegmann, T., Rapid in vivo destruction of semisyngeneic and allogeneic cells by nonimmunized mice as a consequence of nonidentity at H-2, *J. Immunol.,* 118, 2130, 1977.

110. Carlson, G., Taylor, B., Marshall, S., and Greenberg, A., A genetic analysis of natural resistance to nonsyngeneic cells: the role of H-2, *Immunogenetics,* 20, 287, 1984.

111. Klein, G. O., Klein, G., Kiessling, R., and Kärre, K., H-2 associated control of natural cytotoxicity and hybrid resistance against RBL-5, *Immunogenetics,* 6, 561, 1978.

112. Kärre, K., Klein, G. O., Kiessling, R., Argov, S., and Klein, G., The beige model in studies of natural resistance against semisyngeneic, syngeneic and autochtonous tumors in NK cells and other natural effector cells, in *NK Cells and Other Natural Effector Cells,* Herberman, R., Ed., Academic Press, New York, 1982, 1369.

113. Kärre, K., Ljunggren, M., Piontek, G., Kiessling, R., Klein, G., Taniguchi, K., and Gröngberg, A., Activation of cell-mediated immunity by absence or deleted expression of normal cellular gene products, i.e., by "no self" rather than "non self", *Immunobiology,* 167, 43, 1984.

114. Hansson, M., Kärre, K., Kiessling, R., Roder, J., Andersson, B., and Häry, P., Natural NK cell targets in the mouse thymus: characteristics of the sensitivity cell population, *J. Immunol.,* 123, 765, 1979.

115. Stern, P., Gidlund, M., Ön, A., and Wigzell, H., Natural killer cells mediate lysis of embryonal carcinoma cells lacking MHC, *Nature (London),* 285, 341, 1980.

116. Ljunggren, H. and Kärre, K., Host resistance directed selectively against H-2 loss lymphoma variants. Analysis of the mechanisms, *J. Exp. Med.,* 162, 1745, 1985.

117. Becker, S., Kiessling, R., Lee, N., and Klein, G., Modulation of sensitivity to natural killer cell lysis in vitro explantation of a mouse lymphoma, *J. Natl. Cancer Inst.,* 1, 1495, 1978.

118. Piontek, G., Taniguchi, K., Ljunggren, H., Grönberg, A., Kiessling, R., Klein, G., and Karre, K., YAC-1 MHC class I variants reveal an association between decreased NK sensitivity and increased H-2 expression following interferon treatment or in vivo passage, *J. Immunol.,* 135, 4281, 1985.

119. Katzav, S., Segal, S., and Feldman, M., Metastatic capacity of cloned T10 sarcoma cells that differ in H-2 expression: inverse relationship to their immunogenic potency, *J. Natl. Cancer Inst.,* 75, 307, 1985.

120. Taniguchi, K., Kärre, K., and Klein, G., Lung colonization and metastasis by disseminated B16 melanoma cells: H-2 associated control at the level of the host and the tumor cell, in press.

121. Yageeswaran, G., Grönberg, A., Hansson, M., Dalianis, T., Kiessling, R., and Welsh, R., Correlation of gycosphingolipids and sialic acid in YAC-1 lymphoma variants with their sensitivity to natural killer cell mediated lysis, *Int. J. Cancer,* 28, 517, 1981.

122. Gorelik, Elieser, Unpublished observation.

Chapter 4

ALTERATIONS IN NATURAL KILLER CELL ACTIVITY IN TUMOR-BEARING HOSTS

Hugh F. Pross and Malcolm G. Baines

TABLE OF CONTENTS

I. INTRODUCTION

NK cells have been the subject of intense investigation for more than a decade. Although it is now known that NK cells are capable of lysing targets other than tumor cells, the fact that they were first discovered because of their ability to lyse tumor cells has resulted in the major part of the work being directed at determining the role of these cells in defense against malignant disease. It is obvious that there are a number of points in the continuum from neoplastic transformation to the onset of clinically apparent metastatic disease at which an antitumor mechanism could be operative. In a recent chapter in this series, the involvement of NK cells in human malignant disease was reviewed.[1] In this review the NK activity of persons at risk for cancer, NK function during carcinogenesis, NK function in patients with solid tumors, and the possibility of NK surveillance against metastatic disease were discussed. In the present chapter, a more detailed review will be made of one of these topics — the effects of malignant disease on NK cell function and possible mechanisms by which these effects may occur.

II. NK CELL ACTIVITY IN TUMOR-BEARING ANIMALS

There is considerable evidence in the literature that the ability of a transplanted tumor to "take" or to metastasize varies inversely with the NK cell activity of the host. This very simplistic generalization must be modified, however, by stipulating that the tumor cell used in the experiment must be sensitive to NK lysis. Thus, the combination of demonstrable NK activity in the host and tumor susceptibility to NK cells makes it possible to demonstrate an in vivo role for this defense mechanism. These results are well discussed in other chapters in this volume. Unfortunately, there are a number of points at which the system may fail. In animal models low NK activity is the rule rather than the exception, although this activity may frequently be boosted with biological response modifiers such as interferon or IL-2.[2,3] Furthermore, fresh tumor cells are frequently resistant to NK lysis, which also decreases the effectiveness of the system in destroying the tumor in vivo. It is for these reasons that most experiments designed to show the effect of growing tumors on NK activity have involved strains of mice which have detectable NK activity initially, and have used an NK susceptible target, usually the YAC lymphoma cell line, in the assay system. The assumption is made in using experimental systems of this sort that effects seen in an optimal system will also be present in animals with less easily detectable levels of NK activity or in which the tumors are more resistant to being killed.

Among the first experiments designed to determine the effect of tumors on NK cell function were those of Becker and Klein.[4] In these studies, mice with medium and high NK activity were transplanted with methylcholanthrene-induced or Moloney virus-induced sarcomas. The authors also investigated the effect of the presence of human lymphoblastoid cell lines in nude mice on the NK activity of the mice. It was found that in all three systems the NK activity was reduced, although no evidence for suppressor cells was found. The murine sarcoma virus (MSV) system was interesting because MSV-induced tumors regress in these animals so that it was possible to determine NK activity before the appearance of the tumor, during tumor growth, and after regression. It was found that the low NK activity which occurred at the time of maximum tumor size reverted to control levels after the tumor had regressed, suggesting that the effects are short lived and, possibly, operated at the effector level as opposed to causing inhibition at the NK precursor level. Later experiments by others have shown that decreased NK cell activity is by no means invariably observed in tumor-bearing animals. Ehrlich et al.[5] reported that in three tumor systems examined, urethane induced lung adenomas in BALB/c mice, dimethylbenzanthracene (DMBA)-induced tumors in hormonally stimulated BALB/c mice, and mammary tumors in force-bred C3HeB mice, only the NK activity of the mice bearing the DMBA- and the forced breeding-induced tumors was inhibited compared to the controls. Cell mixing experiments of tumor-bearing mouse spleen cells and normal spleen cells showed that the tumor bearing mice contained cells which could suppress NK activity or at least could compete against the target cells for NK cells. Similarly Gerson et al.[6] found that normal levels of splenic NK activity were observed in some tumor-bearing animals, especially young mice, while the splenic NK activity in older tumor bearing mice was extremely low. As in other studies, the results were complicated by the fact that the aging mice had low NK activity in the absence of a tumor. In this study, and a subsequent one involving MSV-induced tumors,[7] depression of NK activity was reversed by depletion of adherent cells. A more detailed discussion of mechanisms of NK suppression in tumor-bearing individuals is given below.

Other experimental systems in which host NK activity has been shown to be suppressed by the presence of tumor include Ehrlich ascites tumors in CBA mice,[8] transplantable and spontaneous mammary adenocarcinoma in C3H mice.[8-10] MH-134 hepatoma in C3H mice,[10] 591 melanoma in DBA mice,[11] B16-F1 and B16-F10 melanoma in C57B1 mice,[12] MBT-2 bladder carcinoma in C3H mice,[13] T241 fibrosarcoma in C3H mice,[14] and Lewis lung carcinoma in C57Bl mice.[10,14-17] A recent study by Lala et al.[8,18] illustrates many of the effects of transplanted and spontaneous tumors on the NK activity of the host. Ehrlich ascites tumor cells and spontaneous mammary tumor cells were injected into syngeneic mice and NK activity was measured at various times. Total spleen NK activity was found to be increased at 3 days, followed by a drop to subnormal levels by 7 days. Single cell NK assays done using spleen cells from the Ehrlich ascites tumor-bearing hosts 10 days to 2 weeks post-transplantation showed no depression of NK-1+ target binding cells (TBC), but a marked decrease in TBC capable of lysing the target, suggesting that the lytic function of the target-binding NK cells was actively impaired. In addition to studying transplanted tumors, Lala et al. also studied NK activity in mice with spontaneous mammary tumors.[8] The authors observed that these mice had progressively depressed NK function while control animals maintained detectable levels which were normal for their age. The enhanced NK activity seen after inoculation of various different tumor types, including spontaneous mammary carcinomas, was not observed in the primary hosts bearing the spontaneous tumors, but this may have been because of the technical difficulties inherent in knowing exactly when such mice should be sacrificed. It is possible that NK stimulation after tumor transplantation is an experimental artifact due to factors such as mycoplasma contamination, fetal calf serum, or in in vivo-derived tumors, contaminating inflammatory cells. Whatever the cause, it was shown by Lala et al.[8] that the stimulated NK cells were capable of preventing tumor take when they were mixed with them in a Winn-type assay.

Several other studies have reported augmented NK activity soon after tumor inoculation. Herberman et al.[19] inoculated young and old Balb/c nude mice with RBL-5 or YC8 ascitic tumor cells and measured splenic NK activity at intervals thereafter. It was found that increased NK activity occurred 24 hr later, but declined by day 3. In a similar study, syngeneic, and allogeneic ascites lymphoma cells were inoculated into conventional and Balb/c nude mice.[20] Again, splenic NK activity increased within 24 hr and declined by the 3rd day. In this study, serum interferon was also measured and it was found that detectable levels of interferon coincided with elevated NK activity. Furthermore, only NK susceptible tumor cells induced interferon in this system, which would argue against the phenomenon being due to an experimental artifact. Slight enhancement of NK activity was also observed by Pollock et al.[17] at day 1 and day 7 after injection of Lewis Lung carcinoma cells followed by marked NK depression at 2 weeks, and by Kärre et al.[21] after the inoculation of leukemia cells to beige and C57B1 litter-mates. These studies indicate that NK stimulation is a potentially protective mechanism by which the host may respond to tumor. On the other hand, the phenomenon is transient and is easily overcome by increasing tumor burden.

Of the many experimental systems which have been used in these studies, the most extensively investigated is the Lewis Lung carcinoma in C57 Black mice. The presence of a large tumor, 2 to 4 weeks post-transplantation, is associated with suppression of NK activity,[10,14-17] which, as mentioned above, may or may not be preceded by a transient increase in splenic cytotoxicity immediately postinoculation.[17] Examination of the effects of the tumor on NK activity in other organs has shown that the system is extremely complex. Kaiserlian et al.[15,16] observed a decrease in splenic NK activity 17 days after the inoculation of Lewis Lung cells, associated with a nonsignificant increase in thymic NK activity. If the tumor was amputated at day 12, splenic NK activity returned to normal values while in the thymus NK cytotoxicity was markedly increased. In these animals the thymus was normal in size, in contrast to the thymic atrophy seen in tumor-bearing mice. NK activity is not usually detected in the thymus of normal animals unless the animal has been treated with hydrocortisone. Treatment of tumor-amputated mice with hydrocortisone resulted in a paradoxical lowering of thymic NK activity compared to the untreated controls. Also, in contrast to normal mice, after hydrocortisone treatment, the TB mouse thymic NK activity was not associated with an increase in peanut agglutinin (PNA) positive cells. Although the target repertoire of these cells was similar to that of splenic NK cells, it was not determined whether the thymic NK cells were phenotypically similar to splenic NK cells. However, the study did point out that experiments in which only splenic NK activity is measured may not reveal the full picture of the effects of the tumor on host NK function. Similarly, suppressed splenic NK activity may not reflect immunosuppression in general. Jones et al.[14] assessed splenic lymphocyte responses to Concanavalin A, lipopolysaccharide, and allogeneic lymphocytes as well as graft-vs.-host reactivity and IL-2 production in Lewis Lung tumor-bearing mice. In these particular experiments, all of these lymphocyte function assays were normal in mice 28 days after tumor implantation, a time point at which marked NK suppression was observed. Although other systems have shown depressed mitogen-responsiveness in parallel with decreased NK activity in tumor-bearing hosts,[11] the data of Jones et al.[14] indicate that tumor-induced suppressor mechanisms may act on the NK cell system independently of other lymphocyte functions. The possible nature of these suppressor mechanisms is discussed below.

III. NK CELL ACTIVITY IN CANCER PATIENTS

The effect of malignant disease on NK function and, conversely, the effect of NK dysfunction on the local and metastatic spread of human solid tumors has been the subject of considerable study in recent years. In 1976 it was first shown by us that patients with advanced metastatic disease had markedly lower NK activity compared to those with local disease, or with no evidence of disease.[22] Shortly thereafter, Takasugi et al. made similar observations[23] and, as can been seen in Table 1, the phenomenon has since been reported by a large number of investigators who have studied many different types of cancer. The details of some of these reports are discussed in the next section. In our original study of 86 patients,[22] the patients with metastatic disease were a biased population, since the majority had advanced disease with liver metastases. To try and assess the biologic and prognostic relevance of low NK activity in cancer patients in general, we embarked on a long-term study of 1600 randomly chosen cancer patients. This study involved four steps.

Table 1
A SUMMARY OF NK FUNCTION IN PATIENTS WITH SOLID TUMORS

Tumor type	Effect on blood NK cell function	
	No change	Decrease
Miscellaneous solid	(29)[b] (30)[c] (37—40)[e]	(22, 23, 31—36)[a] (41)[b] (42, 43)[c] (44)[e]
Melanoma	(45—47)[b] (50)[d]	(48)[a] (49)[c]
Familial melanoma		(51)[b]
Ovary	(52)[c]	(53)[a] (54—58)[c] (59—61)[b]
Cervix, endometrium	(62)[b]	(63—65)[a]
Breast	(29, 66—68, 72—74)[b] (75)[c]	(64, 69—71)[a] (76, 77)[b] (78)[c]
Lung (small cell and nonsmall cell)	(79, 80)[b] (81)[c] (83, 84)[d]	(48)[a] (82)[b] (85—87)[c]
Colon	(88)[c] (89, 90)[d]	(91)[a] (82)[b] (92)[e]
Stomach		(91)[a] (93)[d]
Hepatocellular carcinoma		(94)[e]
Pancreas		(95)[d]
Midgut carcinoid	(96)[c]	
Bladder		(97)[b] (98)[d]
Prostate	(98)[d]	(99, 100)[a] (101)[d]
Primary brain		(102)[d] (29, 103)[e]
Myeloma	(38, 104)[d]	
Malignant lymphoma		(37, 39, 105)[d]
Hodgkin's disease	(106)[d]	(107, 108)[a] (39)[d] (109, 110)[b] (111)[e]
Larynx		(112)[d]
Mycosis fungoides or cutaneous T-cell lymphoma	(113, 114)[e]	(115, 116)[a] (117)[e]

Note: This table includes reports in which there may be duplication in the patients described in different publications by the same author.

[a]   Decrease more evident in advanced disease.
[b]   Mostly nonmetastatic disease reported.
[c]   Mostly advanced local and/or metastatic.
[d]   No stage relationship.
[e]   Stage not reported, mixed, unclear, or not applicable.

1.   The establishment of a logical and reproducible method of NK quantification.[24]
2.   The determination of normal donor NK levels and parameters affecting normal cytotoxic activity.[25]
3.   The actual study and analysis of NK function in cancer patients relative to normal donors.[26]
4.   The long-term follow-up, chart review and data analysis necessary to determine relationships, if any, between NK activity and the various clinical and experimental parameters examined.

At the outset, several decisions were made which could have had some bearing on the results obtained. It was decided to use monocyte-depleted lymphocyte preparations because of the variation in monocyte "contamination" between different individual Ficoll-Isopaque preparations[217] and because of the inhibition of NK activity seen at high effector/target ratios when monocyte-containing mononuclear preparations are used.[27,28] It was also decided that an overnight assay using K562 as the target was the most sensitive method available to detect NK activity and only NK activity.[27,28] The patients studied were suffering from solid tumors such as carcinoma of the lung, endometrium, cervix and ovary, melanoma, Hodgkin's disease, and nonHodgkin's lymphoma. The patients were chosen "randomly" in that blood from all consenting pa-

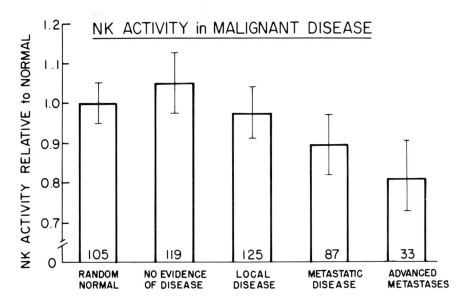

FIGURE 1.   Histogram showing the mean ± SE of the NK activity of patients with various solid tumors relative to normal controls.[26] Each patient was tested from 1 to 34 times for a total of 1455 assays with a median of 3/patient. The geometric mean activity within each disease category was calculated. Prior to performing "*t*" and paired *t*-tests on these data, it was shown that the logged RNK data was normally distributed. The mean RNK for the metastatic and advanced metastatic disease categories are significantly different from the "no evidence of disease" category at $p < 0.04$ and $p < 0.03$ respectively.

tients with those cancers were tested, with the referring physician being unaware of the type of data expected and the investigators being unaware of the diagnosis and condition of the patients. NK assays, lymphocyte markers, natural antibody levels, and immune complexes were determined on most samples and the NK activity was quantitated and expressed relative to normal as described.[26] For this publication, data entry was stopped at 307 patients and a preliminary analysis was done. For each visit the chart was carefully reviewed and the disease status coded as follows: no evidence of disease, local disease, metastatic disease at a single site ± local disease, metastatic disease at multiple sites ± local disease. Several other parameters were recorded which will not be reported here. The results of the analysis are shown in Figure 1. This figure shows the mean NK activity data for each disease category. Within each category, any one patient contributed only one value, which was the mean of all the tests done on that patient (n = 1 − 34, median = 3). The data show that, under the testing conditions described, NK activity was significantly reduced in patients with advanced metastatic disease, but that the actual differences (0.82 ± 0.09 for advanced metastases vs. 1.05 ± 0.07 for patients with no evidence of disease) were not marked, and certainly not as great as reported by us for patients with liver metastases, or by others using unfractionated mononuclear cells (the majority of papers referred to in Table 1). We feel that the use of purified lymphocytes, the overnight assay, careful quantification, and some degree of investigator "blindness" account for the data observed and support its validity. Our present efforts are directed at completing the entry of data from patients, who have already been tested, in order to have enough patients within the different disease and stage classifications for accurate analysis. A major aim of the work will be to correlate mean NK activity with survival time from diagnosis, with survival time from the test data and with the time from "no evidence of disease", or "local disease", to the diagnosis of metastases at different sites. Hopefully, this analysis will contribute to our under-

Table 2
POSSIBLE MECHANISMS OF NK INHIBITION IN
MALIGNANT DISEASE

In situ sequestration of NK cells.
Immune complex blockade of Fc receptors.
Blockade of NK recognition receptors by "antigen" or immune complexes.
NK inhibitory factors.
Suppressor T-cells.
Suppressor monocytes/macrophages.
Inhibition of positive regulators (IL-2, IFN).
Stimulation of negative regulators (prostaglandins).

standing of the relevance of NK activity in vivo and will determine the value of assessing NK activity as a prognostic variable in cancer patients.

IV. THE MECHANISM OF NK INHIBITION IN TUMOR-BEARING INDIVIDUALS

Although our own data show a minimal, but significant, reduction in NK activity in patients with cancer, and as can be seen on Table 1, several investigators have observed no significant reduction in NK activity in cancer patients, there is still considerable evidence from animal models and many other patient studies that the presence of a tumor in the host has an inhibitory effect on NK activity. The mechanism of the effect still remains to be determined, but a number of possible mechanisms have been investigated. Most of the studies have been interpreted in light of our present concepts of NK regulation, i.e., that NK cells are positively regulated by interferon and IL-2 and negatively regulated by prostaglandins. The regulation of NK cells has been reviewed extensively by Herberman[118,119] and Kimber and Moore[120] and will not be discussed in depth here. In addition to the regulatory effects of these molecules on NK activity, the individual animal or person has a certain "endogenous" level of NK activity which is genetically determined. It is well-established that certain strains of mice are high or low NK-activity strains[121] while in man, baseline NK function is fairly stable for a particular individual relative to the normal mean.[25] In man, normal adult levels of NK activity are maintained into old age[25,122-124] whereas in mice NK activity becomes almost undetectable after 5 or 6 months of age, depending on the strain.[121] It has been suggested that this low NK activity in old mice is due to a heightened sensitivity to the inhibitory effects of prostaglandins resulting in low endogenous and interferon stimulated activity.[125] In view of the complexity of normal NK regulatory mechanisms, it is not surprising that the mechanism whereby tumor growth affects NK function has also proven to be extremely complex, since inhibitory factors may act directly on NK cells or NK precursors, or the inhibitory effects may be indirectly mediated by perturbations in the NK regulatory network (Table 2).

Because the majority of NK studies in tumor-bearing hosts involve peripheral blood mononuclear cells (in man) or spleen cells (in animals), it is possible that the observed decrease in NK activity is due to NK cell migration to the tumor site or to the draining lymph nodes. Studies on the NK activity of malignant effusion or tumor-infiltrating lymphocytes (TIL) do not support this hypothesis, however. Most, but not all, studies have shown NK activity to be absent or very low in draining nodes,[76,126-130] effusions,[54,58,59,61,85] or at the tumor site.[6,7,55,72,102,126,127,129,130-134] This is partly due to an inhibition of *in situ* NK cell activity since it has been possible to enrich for functional NK cells by Percoll gradient centrifugation from ascites fluids and tumor infiltrating lymphocytes.[55,61,134,135] The frequency of LGL or NK marker-bearing cells *in situ* is low,[55,134] however, and it is difficult to conceive that this level of NK cell infiltration would have any impact on a cell population which makes up 1 to 3% of peripheral blood lymphocytes.

Although intratumor NK cell sequestration may not be the mechanism by which NK cell activity is reduced in peripheral blood, there is some evidence that the frequency of NK cells in the blood of cancer patients is reduced. Balch et al.[136] showed a significant decrease in HNK-1 positive cells in 247 patients with a variety of solid tumors. Significant differences were found in patients with carcinoma of the colon, lung and head and neck, but not in melanoma or sarcoma patients. The most significant differences were seen between carcinoma of the colon patients (9.7%, n = 49) and controls (15.5%, n = 146). There were no differences between different stages of the same tumor. In contrast to the age-independence of functional NK assays, it was found that age-matching of patients and controls was essential to demonstrating these differences. Although not all HNK-1 positive cells are active NK cells, the data were interpreted as indicating a decrease in LGL frequency in the patient population. Hajto and Lanzrein[71] also described a reduction in LGL in advanced breast cancer and Tanaka et al.[93] reported a decrease in target binding cells in patients with gastric cancer. Both of these observations may reflect a decrease in NK cell frequency in peripheral blood. Similarly, Gastl et al.[44] noted a decrease in the frequency of LGL in the PBL of patients with solid tumors (2 to 20% with a mean of 8% for cancer patients vs. 5 to 29% with a mean of 14% for normals). The proportional reduction in cytotoxicity between normals and cancer patients was greater than that seen for the LGL counts, suggesting a functional defect as well as a frequency defect. It is difficult to determine whether this conclusion is valid, however, since the proportional change in NK activity was calculated using percent chromium release at one E/T ratio, as opposed to using lytic units.[24]

In contrast to these data, Steinhauer et al.,[34] using the single cell cytotoxic assay and kinetic analysis, demonstrated that the frequency of NK cells in patients with breast cancer was normal, while recycling capacity was reduced. Our own studies[217] also failed to show a reduction in NK cell frequency to account for diminished NK activity in cancer patients. In these studies Fc receptor positive non-B, non-T-lymphocytes were enumerated and the results were correlated with NK activity. No correlation was found between the percentage of these cells (which include virtually all NK cells) and relative NK cytotoxicity, implying that the NK defect is one of function and not frequency.

Because NK cells are Fc receptor positive and possess some type of receptor for the tumor cell target structure, it is possible that immune complexes and/or soluble "antigens" could have an inhibitory effect on NK activity in the tumor-bearing host.[137] In vitro, it is well established that Fc receptor blockade with immune complexes inhibits NK activity,[138-141] even though the Fc receptor is not necessary for NK function.[139,140,142] However, attempts to correlate serum or effusion immune complex levels with NK activity have shown no direct correlation, either in cancer patients[143] or animal models.[9] The possibility that NK inhibition in tumor-bearing individuals can be attributed to recognition receptor binding by soluble tumor-derived "antigens" has not been extensively investigated. Early in vitro work by Roder et al.[144] showed that nonadherent splenocyte-target cell binding could be inhibited by isolated target structures from the YAC cell line, the NK-sensitive cell line most commonly used in murine NK experiments. In these studies 3 glycoproteins of mol wt 130,000, 160,000, and 240,000 were isolated.[144] The molecules were separable from the Moloney lymphoma cell surface antigen, gp39, gp71, and H2, and were "specific" in inhibitory effect in that binding to YAC was inhibited by extracts from NK sensitive cell lines, but not with material from resistant lines. Alloimmune CTL-target binding was not inhibited by any of the molecules isolated. Subsequent investigations by many laboratories have implicated glycoproteins and glycolipids as target molecules in human,[145-147] and murine[148-151] systems. Inhibition of NK activity is greatly enhanced if the inhibitor is asialated[148,150,152] and the sugar residues in these molecules play a major role in causing inhibition.[153-157]

In theory, release of these or similar glycosylated molecules into the serum or effusion fluid of tumor-bearing individuals could cause inhibition of NK activity in vivo, but there is little evidence for or against this hypothesis. Inhibition of normal NK activity has been observed with sera or effusion fluids from tumor-bearing patients[60,158,159] and animals[9,160,161] in some but not all experiments.[94] In those studies where attempts have been made to characterize the phenomenon, the source of the inhibitor has been the nontumor lymphoid cells or macrophages, suggesting a regulatory molecule as opposed to recognition receptor blockade.[158,161,163] There is considerable evidence that prostaglandins may be implicated as the suppressor molecule (see below), but Zigelboim et al.,[60,158,161] in studies of cells from rats and humans, suggest that a nonprostaglandin NK inhibitory substance, termed NK-IS, is produced by nonadherent peritoneal exudate cells. NK-IS is a low molecular weight, protease resistant substance capable of inhibiting rat, mouse, and human NK activity, but not murine or human CTL.[161] It is not released by tumor cells and its production by PE cells is not inhibited by indomethacin. These interesting observations await confirmation by other investigators.

Suppressor T-cells have long been suggested as playing a role in the specific and nonspecific immunosuppression of malignancy (as well as other diseases).[164,165] Zoller and Wigzell[166] have described a Helix pomatia receptor positive Thy-1-positive (in the mouse), Ly-1 and Ly-2 positive (in the rat), Ig negative, FcR negative nonadherent lymphocyte in normal rats, and mice capable of suppressing NK activity. The cell is similar to the NK-inhibitory cell which is activated by *Corynebacterium parvum*.[167] To the best of our knowledge this suppressor cell has not been shown to be activated in tumor-bearing mice or rats. In man, however, Tarkannen et al.[168] have described a small, high density FcR positive NK suppressor cell in 9/55 normal donors and 1/25 cancer patients. These cells could be activated by immune complexes and were identifiable in a greater proportion of individuals after PBL fractionation. An FcuR HNK-1 positive T marker-negative suppressor lymphocyte has also been documented by D'Amore and Golub.[169] This cell, different from that of Tarkannen et al.,[168] was generated in mixed lymphocyte culture reactions and inhibited both NK- and MLC-generated NK activity. However, as was the case with murine lymphocytic NK-suppressor cells, there is no evidence that these cells are responsible for tumor-induced NK suppression.

Monocyte-macrophage suppressor cells have also been implicated as being NK-suppressive. These experiments are discussed below in the section dealing with prostaglandin-induced NK inhibition.

Alterations in the balance between the interleukins, interferons, and prostaglandins must also play an important role in tumor-induced NK-inhibition. NK cells are stimulated directly by interferons to become more actively cytolytic via a combination of mechanisms involving increased recycling and target-binding capacity, increased NK frequency and a somewhat broader target repertoire.[2,170-174] Many studies have examined the ability of NK cells from cancer patients[32,58,63,78,95,105,108] or tumor-bearing animals[11,13,18,160,175] to respond to interferon and, in general, the observation has been that low NK activity is associated with poor responsiveness to interferon. The phenomenon is difficult to quantify and is dependent on the type of cancer or animal tumor being studied, the degree of tumor burden, and the type of interferon used. It has been shown that tumor cells can induce interferon production by NK (and other) cells[20,176] and it is possible that constant exposure to interferon in vivo can lead to an interferon-refractory state analogous to that seen in patients reveiving interferon therapy.[30,177] On the other hand, strong interferon inducers, such as virus-modified tumor cell extracts (in patients with ovarian cancer[58]) or vaccinia infection (in DBA/2 mice bearing melanoma tumors[11]) can overcome the low NK of the tumor-bearing host, an observation which may be relevant to the clinical application of biological response modifiers.

A series of publications by Kadish et al.[32,34,63,78,178] has examined in depth the relationship between malignant disease, NK activity, and interferon. The data are interesting in that several different aspects of the IFN-NK interaction have been investigated. The initial paper from this group[32] dealt with the NK activity of 51 patients with several different solid epithelial tumors, both localized and advanced. PBL NK activity was suppressed in advanced disease, but pretreatment of the PBL with interferon-α or Newcastle Disease Virus (NDV) enhanced the cytotoxicity of most, although not all, of the low NK donors. In spite of the fact that NK activity was low and only partially restored with interferon, it was found that NDV or K562 induced interferon production in all PBL preparations, supporting the conclusion that the NK defect does not lie at the level of IFN production. A similar failure of responsiveness to IFN was observed in patients with advanced cervical cancer[63] and other solid tumors.[33] In a subsequent study, Steinhauer et al.[34] applied single cell cytotoxicity and kinetic assay techniques to the analysis of the defect. In this study, it was found that the maximum killing of the patients' cells (Vmax) was reduced, while NK frequency remained normal, suggesting that the NK defect is at the level of the recycling capability. A similar recycling defect was postulated to explain the NK defect of lung tumor-infiltrating lymphocytes by Moy et al.[134] In this study, 15 TIL preparations were compared with PBL from the same patients with respect to Vmax, target-binding cells and lytic target-binding cells. Vmax was significantly reduced, while both PBL and TIL had similar proportions of target-binding lymphocytes and lytic cells. The proportions of cells with the NK-inclusive markers HNK-1 and B73.1 were also similar. Together these papers suggest that, at a certain tumor burden, local NK inhibitory effects are exerted on the systemic PBL NK population as a whole. Recently Steinhauer et al.[78,178] have extended their studies to an investigation of the role of NK cytotoxic factor (NKCF) in this phenomenon. In confirmation of Wright and Bonavida[179] NKCF was found to be released from normal PBL cocultured with the NK target K562.[178] NKCF was consistently found in association with interferon-α but not vice versa, and anti-interferon abrogated NKCF production. In 23 patients with advanced malignant disease, PBL from 15 showed defective ability to produce NKCF and 10 of these were deficient in interferon production.[78] PBL from 8 of the patients were also deficient in NK activity vs. K562. These data suggest that tumor-induced NK-inhibitory mechanisms affecting NK cytokine and NKCF production can be detected before overall diminution in lytic activity is detected. This mechanism of NK inhibition could be acting in addition to a recycling defect, and contributing to it because of reduced local IFN concentrations, or alternatively, the recycling defect could be an apparent defect only, caused by insufficient NKCF being released from the target-binding NK cell to cause lysis before the cell moves to another target. An interesting speculation provoked by these data is that other NK-derived cytokines[180] could be inhibited by advanced malignant disease, resulting in defects in the postulated immunoregulatory functions of these cells.[181] At present this is a relatively unexplored area.

Although interferon is the most extensively studied NK stimulatory molecule, IL-2 is also fundamental to maintaining optimum NK frequency and activity. IL-2 also has direct stimulatory effect on NK cells,[3,182] and, is probably required for the generation of mature NK cells from NK-precursors.[183-185] IL-2 is produced by stimulated T-cells and IL-2 production is dependent on accessory cell-derived IL-1.[186,187] Although there is very little data in the literature relating NK, interleukins, and malignant disease, it is reasonable to assume that factors which affect interleukin production will in turn affect NK activity.

The interleukins have been assessed in a variety of types of cancer, both in man and animals. Ravikumar et al.[188] observed a significant reduction in both IL-1 and IL-2 production from peripheral blood mononuclear cells in rats bearing experimetnal colon carcinomas. The decrease was noted while the tumor was still localized and became profound as the tumour progressed. In this model, interleukin inhibition reflected tumor burden, with the effects being reversed if the tumors were removed or effectively treated with immunotherapy. The type of immunotherapy, i.e. irradiated tumor cells, butanol-extracted tumor cells or antigen-containing liposomes did not affect the suppressive activity of recurrent tumors. On the other hand, successful immunotherapy was associated with recovery of interleukin production. Whether the success of the immunotherapy was due to the recovery of interleukin production, as opposed to IL-2 production being merely a reflection of decreased tumor load, is a possibility which merits further investigation. An interesting peripheral observation in this work was that repetitive ether anesthesia and bleeding of the control tumor-free animals also caused some decrease in interleukin production. Similar effects may be responsible for the transient (5 to 7 days) decrease in NK activity seen in individuals undergoing major surgery,[52,68,74,189-191] a phenomenon which has been reported to be adherent cell dependent.[74,91]

The effect of tumor burden on IL-2 production has also been reported by Kedar et al.,[192] in Balb/c, C57 Bl/6 and C3H mice bearing various different epithelial and lyphoid tumors and by Burger et al.[193] in Balb/c mice bearing fibrosarcomas. Both groups reported that IL-2 inhibition was apparently mediated by an Lyt-2 positive suppressor T-cell. Removal of this cell population markedly increased IL-2 production beyond that expected on the basis of the enrichment of the remaining cells. Kedar et al.[192] found that removal of phagocytes from the cell preparations, or treatment with indomethacin, also increased IL-2 production, implicating macrophages and prostaglandins as being active in suppression. Interestingly, addition of tumor cells in vitro did not suppress Con-A-induced IL-2 production by the splenocytes. In contrast to these data, Jones et al.[14] observed normal IL-2 production in C57Bl mice 2 to 4 weeks after implantation with the Lewis Lung carcinoma. However, as discussed above, NK activity in the system was suppressed.

Defective IL-2 production by PBL from cancer patients has also been observed in several studies[42,43,194-197] and there appears to be little controversy as to the relationship between tumor burden and inhibition. Rey et al.[43] related the IL-2 inhibition to the defective NK activity seen in cancer patients, supporting the hypothesis that the interleukin defect may be the primary cause of the NK defect. Some investigators[195,198,199] although not all[194] have also reported defective IL-1 production in cancer patients.

As in other systems, the mechanism of interleukin inhibition is unknown. Hersey et al.[196] and Fontana et al.[195] documented the release of IL-2 inhibitory factors from cultured melanoma and glioblastoma cells respectively. The melanoma-derived factor inhibited PHA-induced IL-2 production, but had no effect on IL-1 production or the activity of preformed IL-2. The glioblastoma-derived factor, similar in many respects to neuroblast growth inhibition factor, inhibited IL-2 induced proliferation and the two factors are obviously different from each other. It is not known what the effect is of these factors on NK cell function per se and, conversely, studies showing the presence of inhibitory factors on NK activity[200,201] did not examine effects on interleukin production. Many papers have dealt with the production of biologically active factors by cultured tumor cells and a detailed discussion of the field is beyond the scope of this review.

There is considerable evidence that adherent cells and/or prostaglandins are major mediators of the suppression of NK activity in both normal[7,119,125,163,175,202-213] and tumor-bearing hosts,[6,7,18,31,102,103,214] whether by inhibition of interleukin production or by direct action on the NK cells themselves. Lala et al. have recently described the "inactivation" of NK cells in mice bearing several different types of tumor (see above[8]). In an elegant series of experiments to determine the mechanism of the phenomenon, Parhar and Lala[18] found that mixing of tumor-bearing spleen cells with normal spleen cells resulted in no effect on NK activity at the effector cell level, but caused marked suppression if the cells were co-cultured for 20 hr. The suppression could be abrogated by incorporating indomethacin in the cultures, suggesting that the suppressive effects were due to prostaglandins, and the suppressor cells were phagocytic, Mac-1 positive, adherent, and morphologically macrophages. This NK suppressor mechanism may be similar to that shown by Brunda et al.[175] and by Zoller and Matzka[163] in normal murine PE cells, but not in spleen cells. In the latter experiments, coincubation of tumor targets with the macrophages resulted in the production of a suppressive factor, although whether this was prostaglandin was not determined. As was observed by Parhar and Lala,[18] the adherent suppressor cell of Brunda et al.[175] also acted at the pre-NK effector stage and a period of co-culture was required.

Adherent cells have also been shown to be NK-suppressive in cancer patients. In three reports of patients with advanced extracranial tumors[31] and primary intracranial malignancies[102,103] it was found that depletion of adherent cells resulted in augmentation of NK function, an observation which was attributed to hyperactivation of monocyte regulatory function.[103] Adherent cell depletion also augmented NK activity of malignant peritoneal or pleural effusion cells in some,[85,214] but not all[54,131] reports. These cells are, of course, different from the nonadherent PE cells responsible for the production of the suppressive factors described by Zigelboim, Lichtenstein et al.[60,161,162] and others[215] and it was not established whether or not similar suppressive factors could be identified. Nor was it determined whether the adherent cell effects were in fact mediated by prostaglandins in these studies.

However, a recent study by Fulton et al.[68] did attempt to relate prostaglandins and NK activity with negative results. In this study PBL NK activity was measured in women undergoing surgery for primary breast cancer. Although a negative correlation was observed between NK activity and maximum tumor diameter, no correlation was seen with other standard prognostic variables, or the tumor's content of PGE_2 and PGF_2. The lack of correlation between tumor prostaglandin and NK activity may be due to the inability of local prostaglandin to influence systemic NK cells and to the comparative lack of activity of PGF_2 in inhibiting NK function.

V. THE PROGNOSTIC SIGNIFICANCE OF LOW NK ACITIVTY IN TUMOR-BEARING HOSTS

Several chapters in this volume have documented the role of NK cells in preventing the induction of tumors, the initial "take" of transplanted tumor cells and the spread of metastatic foci from the primary tumor. The implication from these experimental data is that low NK activity is relevant to the ability of the animal or patient with cancer to survive the disease. Whether this is so or not has not been established. Hersey et al.[216] failed to show any correlation between NK activity after surgery and recurrence free period or death from melanoma in 212 stage I and 85 stage II patients. In contrast to this result, Mackay et al.[75] showed that, over a 4 year period of follow-up of patients with axillary node-positive breast cancer treated with surgery and 1 year of adjuvant chemotherapy, NK activity 1 year after the start of chemotherapy was significantly lower in 14 to 30 patients who developed recurrent disease than it was in the 16 who remained disease-free. In a somewhat similar study of patients treated with chemotherapy for lung cancer, Saijo et al.[86] noted that recovery of NK activity of chemotherapy correlated well with the effect of chemotherapy. On the other hand, as mentioned previously, Fulton et al.[68] found no correlation between PBL NK levels of breast cancer patients and prognostically-relevant variables such as the number of positive axillary nodes or tumor grade. They did observe a negative correlation with tumor size, however. These latter studies did not determine whether or not NK levels themselves were a prognostic factor which yielded information not available using conventional or laboratory techniques.

Many laboratories, including our own, have accumulated extensive data on NK levels in patients with cancer. Although the process is tedious, it should be possible to go back to the charts on these patients to determine whether or not NK activity has any relevance to survival in cancer. Until this has been done on a sufficiently large number of patients, with their course followed for at least 5 years, the question of relevance will remain unanswered.

VI. SUMMARY

In this chapter we have attempted to review data from human and animal studies on the effect of malignant disease on NK function. In general, NK activity is suppressed in patients or animals bearing advanced or metastatic tumors. Many hypotheses have been proposed to account for this phenomenon. Perhaps the most tenable hypothesis, in the light of current evidence and our knowledge of normal NK-regulatory mechanisms, is that the presence of the tumor results in aberrations of normal NK-regulatory mechanisms, i.e. inhibition of the positive regulatory action of IL-2 and/or stimulation of the negative regulatory action of prostaglandins. There is considerable evidence in support of this hypothesis. The significance of low NK function in malignant disease remains to be established.

ACKNOWLEDGMENTS

We would like to thank Mrs. Mabel Chau, Mrs. Pamela Bandy-Dafoe, and Miss Ingrid Louwman for excellent technical assitance, and Ms. Christine Jackson for typing the manuscript. The work was supported by grants from the Medical Research Council of Canada, the National Cancer Institute of Canada, and the Ontario Cancer Treatment and Research Foundation. H.F. Pross was a Career Scientist of the Ontario Cancer Treatment and Research Foundation.

REFERENCES

1. Pross, H., The involvement of natural killer cells in human malignant disease, in *The Immunobiology of Natural Killer Cells,* Lotzova, E., and Herberman, R. B., Eds., CRC Press, Boca Raton, Fla., 1985.
2. Trinchieri, G. and Santoli, D., Enhancement of human natural killer cell activity by interferon, *J. Immunol.,* 120, 1845, 1978.
3. Trinchieri, G., Matsumoto-Kobayashi, M., Clark, S. C., Seehra, J., London, L., and Perussia, B., Response of resting human peripheral blood natural killer cells to interleukin 2, *J. Exp. Med.,* 160, 1147, 1984.
4. Becker, S. and Klein, E., Decreased 'natural killer' effect in tumor-bearing mice and its relation to the immunity against oncornavirus-determined cell surface antigens, *Eur. J. Immunol.,* 6, 892, 1976.
5. Ehrlich, R., Efrati, M., Bar-Eyal, A., Wollberg, M., Schiby, G., Ran, M., and Witz, I., Natural cellular reactivities mediated by splenocytes from mice bearing three types of primary tumor, *Int. J. Cancer,* 26, 315, 1980.

6. Gerson, J., Tagliabue, A., and Herberman, R., Systemic and in situ natural killer activity in transplanted and spontaneous mammary tumors in C3H/HEN mice, *J. Reticuloendothel. Soc.,* 29, 15, 1981.

7. Gerson, J., Varesio, L., and Herberman, R., Systemic and in situ natural killer and suppressor cell activities in mice bearing progressively growing murine sarcoma-virus-induced tumors, *Int. J. Cancer,* 27, 243, 1981.

8. Lala, P., Santer, V., Libenson, H., and Parhar, R., Changes in the host natural killer cell population in mice during tumor development. I. Kinetics and in vivo significance, *Cell. Immunol.,* in press, 1985.

9. Nair, P., Fernandes, G., Onoe, K., Day, N., and Good, R., Inhibition of effector cell functions in natural killer cell activity and antibody-dependent cellular cytotoxicity in mice by normal and cancer sera, *Int. J. Cancer,* 25, 667, 1980.

10. Ono, M., Tanaka, N., and Orita, K., Dissociation of natural killer activity and antibody-dependent cellular cytotoxicity in spleen cells of tumor bearing mice, *Acta Med. Okayama,* 37, 367, 1983.

11. Byrne, J., Soloski, M., and Holowczak, J., Immune responses of DBA/2 mice bearing melanoma tumors: cell-mediated immune responses after challenge with vaccinia virus, *Cancer Immunol. Immunother.,* 16, 81, 1983.

12. Ehrlich, R., Smorodinsky, N., Efrati, M., Yaakubowicz, M., and Witz, I., B16 melanoma development, NK activity, cytostasis and natural antibodies in 3 and 12 month old mice, *Br. J. Cancer,* 49, 769, 1984.

13. Morales, A. and Pang, A., The effect of tumor burden on the modulation of natural killer cell activity, *J. Urol.,* 131, 1229, 1984.

14. Jones, C., Lee, C., Skinner, W., Koyama, P., and Prescott, D., Absence of generalized immunosuppression in C57BL/6J mice implanted with Lewis T241 fibrosarcoma or Lewis lung carcinoma, *Cancer Immunol. Immunother.,* 18, 82, 1984.

15. Kaiserlian, D., Savino, W., and Bach, J., Studies of the thymus in mice bearing the Lewis lung carcinoma. I. Thymic natural killer activity in 3LL tumor-bearing mice, *Cell. Immunol.,* 80, 187, 1983.

16. Kaiserlian, D., Savino, W., and Dardenne, M., Studies of the thymus in mice bearing the Lewis lung carcinoma. II. Modulation of thymic natural killer activity by Thymulin (FTS-ZN) and the antimetastatic effect of zinc, *Clin. Immunol. Immunopathol.,* 28, 192, 1983.

17. Pollock, R., Babcock, G., Romsdhal, M., and Nishioka, K., Surgical stress-mediated suppression of murine natural killer cell cytotoxicity, *Cancer Res.,* 44, 3888, 1984.

18. Parhar, R. and Lala, P., Changes in the host natural killer cell population in mice during tumor development. II. The mechanism of suppression of NK activity, *Cell. Immunol.,* in press, 1985.

19. Herberman, R., Nunn, M., Holden, H., Staal, S., and Djeu, J., Augmentation of natural cytotoxic reactivity of mouse lymphoid cells against syngeneic and allogeneic target cells, *Int. J. Cancer,* 19, 555, 1977.

20. Djeu, J., Huang, K., and Herberman, R., Augmentation of mouse natural killer activity and induction of interferon by tumor cells in vivo, *J. Exp. Med.,* 151, 781, 1980.

21. Kärre, K., Klein, G., Kiessling, R., Klein, G., and Roder, J., In vitro NK-activity and in vivo resistance to leukemia: studies of beige, beige/nude and wild-type hosts on C57BL background, *Int. J. Cancer,* 26, 789, 1980.

22. Pross, H. and Baines, M., Spontaneous human lymphocyte-mediated cytotoxicity against tumor target cells. I. The effect of malignant disease, *Int. J. Cancer,* 18, 593, 1976.

23. Takasugi, M., Ramseyer, A., and Takasugi, J., Decline of natural nonselective cell-mediated cytotoxicity in patients with tumor progression, *Cancer Res.,* 37, 413, 1977.

24. Pross, H. F., Baines, M. G., Rubin, P., Shragge, P., and Patterson, M., Spontaneous human lymphocyte-mediated cytotoxicity against tumour target cells. IX. Quantitation of natural killer cell activity, *J. Clin. Immunol.,* 1, 51, 1981.

25. Pross, H. and Baines, M., Studies of human natural killer cells. I. In vivo parameters affecting normal cytotoxic function, *Int. J. Cancer,* 29, 383, 1982.

26. Pross, H. F. and Maroun, J. A., The standardization of NK cell assays for use in studies of biological response modifiers, *J. Immunol. Methods,* 68, 235, 1984.

27. Jondal, M. and Pross, H., Surface markers on human B- and T-lymphocytes. VI. Cytotoxicity against cell lines as a functional marker for lymphocyte subpopulations, *Int. J. Cancer,* 15, 596, 1975.

28. Pross, H., Callewaert, D., and Rubin, P., Assays for NK cell cytotoxicity; their values and pitfalls, in *The Immunology of Natural Killer Cells,* Lotzova, E. and Herberman, R., Eds., CRC Press, Boca Raton, Fla., in press, 1984.

29. Gerson, J., Systemic and in situ natural killer activity in tumor-bearing mice and patients with cancer, in *Natural Cell-Mediated Immunity against Tumors,* Herberman, R. B., Ed., Academic Press, New York, 1980, p 1047.

30. Maluish, A., Ortaldo, J., Conlon, J., Sherwin, S., Leavitt, R., Strong, D., Weirnik, P., Oldham, R., and Herberman, R., Depression of natural killer cytotoxicity after in vivo administration of recombinant leukocyte interferon, *J. Immunol.*, 131, 503, 1983.

31. De Boer, K. P., Braun, D., and Harris, J., Natural cytotoxicity and antibody dependent cytotoxicity in solid tumor cancer patients: regulation by adherent cells, *Clin. Immunol. Immunopathol.*, 23, 133, 1982.

32. Kadish, A., Doyle, A., Steinhauer, E., and Ghossein, N., Natural cytotoxicity and interferon production in human cancer: deficient natural killer activity and normal interferon production in patients with advanced disease, *J. Immunol.*, 127, 1817, 1981.

33. Kadish, A. and Ghossein, N., Natural cytotoxicity in patients undergoing radiation therapy, *Am. J. Clin. Oncol.*, 6, 53, 1983.

34. Steinhauer, E., Doyle, A., Reed, J., and Kadish, A., Defective natural cytotoxicity in patients with cancer: normal number of effector cells but decreased recycling capacity in patients with advanced disease, *J. Immunol.*, 129, 2255, 1982.

35. Oldham, R., Djeu, J., Cannon, G., Siwarski, D., and Herberman, R., Cellular microcytotoxicity in human tumor systems: analysis of results, *J. Natl. Cancer Inst.*, 55, 1305, 1975.

36. Menon, M. and Stefani, S., Lymphocyte mediated natural cytotoxicity in neoplasia, *Oncology*, 35, 63, 1978.

37. Lipinski, M., Dokhelar, M -C., and Tursz, T., NK cell activity in patients with high risk for tumors and in patients with cancer, in *NK Cells and Other Natural Effector cells*, Herberman, R. B., Ed., Academic Press, New York, 1982, p 1183.

38. Einhorn, S., Blomgren, H., Strander, H., and Wasserman, J., Influence of human interferon-a therapy on cytotoxic functions of blood lymphocytes. Studies on lectin-dependent cellular cytotoxicity, antibody-dependent cellular cytotoxicity, and antural killer cell activity, *Cancer Immunol. Immunother.*, 16, 77, 1983.

39. Tursz, T., Dokhelar, M., Lipinski, M., and Amiel, J., Low natural killer cell activity in patients with malignant lymphoma, *Cancer*, 50, 2333, 1982.

40. Lucero, M., Fridman, W., Provost, M., Billardon, C., Pouillart, P., Dumont, J., and Falcoff, E., Effect of various interferons on the spontaneous cytotoxicity exerted by lymphocytes from normal and tumor-bearing patients, *Cancer Res.*, 41, 294, 1981.

41. Catalona, W., Ratliff, T., and McCool, R., Discordance among cell-mediated cytolytic mechanisms in cancer patients: importance of the assay system, *J. Immunol.*, 122, 1009, 1979.

42. Rey, A., Klein, B., Zagury, D., Thierry, C., and Serrou, B., Diminished interleukin-2 activity production in cancer patients bearing solid tumors and its relationship with natural killer cells, *Immunol. Lett.*, 6, 175, 1983.

43. Rey, A., Klein, B., Rucheton, M., Caraux, J., Zagury, D., Thierry, C., and Serrou, B., Human autologous rosettes. IV. Their relation with interleukin 2 activity production and natural killer cells in cancer patients, *Cell. Immunol.*, 86, 155, 1984.

44. Gastl, G., Niederwieser, D., Marth, C., Huber, H., Egg, D., Schuler, G., Margreiter, R., Braunsteiner, H., and Huber, C., Human large granular lymphocytes and their relationship to natural killer cell activity in various disease states, *Blood*, 64, 288, 1984.

45. Kristensen, E., A comparative study of natural cytotoxicity and the leukocyte migration inhibition in human melanoma stages I and II, *J. Cancer Res. Clin. Oncol.*, 96, 181, 1980.

46. Kristensen, E., Brandslund, I., Nielsen, H., and Svehag, S. -E., Prognostic value of assays for circulating immune complexes and natural cytotoxicity in malignant skin melanoma (Stages I and II), *Cancer Immunol. Immunother.*, 9, 31, 1980.

47. Hersey, P., Hobbs, A., Edwards, A., McCarthy, W., and McGovern, V., Relationship between natural killer cell activity and histological features of lymphocyte infiltration and partial regression of the primary tumor in melanoma patients, *Cancer Res.*, 42, 363, 1982.

48. Sibbitt, W., Bankhurst, A., Jumonville, A., Saiki, J., Saiers, J., and Doberneck, R., Defects in natural killer cell activity and interferon response in human lung carcinoma and malignant melanoma, *Cancer Res.*, 44, 852, 1984.

49. Thatcher, N., Swindell, R., and Drowther, D., Effects of Corynebacterium parvum and BCG therapy on immune parameters in patients with disseminated melanoma. A sequential study over 28 days. II. Changes in non-specific (NK, K and T Cell) lymphocytoxicity and delayed hypersensitivity skin reactions, *Clin. Exp. Immunol.*, 35, 171, 1979.

50. Yanagawa, E., Uchida, A., Kokoschka, E., and Micksche, M., Natural cytotoxicity of lymphocytes and monocytes and its augmentation by OK432 in melanoma patients, *Cancer Immunol. Immunother.*, 16, 131, 1984.

51. Hersey, P., Edwards, A., Honeyman, M., and McCarthy, W., Low natural killer cell activity in familial melanoma patients and their relatives, *Br. J. Cancer*, 40, 113, 1979.

52. Lukomska, B., Olszewski, W., Engeset, A., and Kolstad, P., The effect of surgery and chemotherapy on blood NK cell activity in patients with ovarian cancer, *Cancer*, 51, 465, 1983.

53. Pross, H. and Baines, M., Natural Killer Cells in Tumour-Bearing Patients, in *Natural Cell-Mediated Immunity Against Tumors,* Herberman, R. B., Ed., Academic Press, New York, 1980, p. 1063.

54. Allavena, P., Introna, M., Mangioni, C., and Mantovani, A., Inhibition of natural killer activity by tumor-associated lymphoid cells from ascites ovarian carcinomas, *J. Natl. Cancer Inst.*, 67, 319, 1981.

55. Introna, M., Allavena, P., Biondi, A., Colombo, N., Villa, A., and Mantovani, A., Defective natural killer activity within human ovarian tumors: low numbers of morphologically defined effectors present in situ, *J. Natl. Cancer Inst.*, 70, 21, 1983.

56. Allavena, P., Introna, M., Sessa, C., Mangioni, C., and Mantovani, A., Interferon effect on cytotoxicity of peripheral blood and tumor-associated lymphocytes against human ovarian carcinoma cells, *J. Natl. Cancer Inst.*, 68, 555, 1982.

57. Colotta, F., Rambaldi, A., Colombo, N., Tabacchi, L., Introna, M., and Mantovani, A., Effect of a streptococcal preparation (OK432) on natural killer activity of tumour-associated lymphoid cells in human ovarian carcinoma and on lysis of fresh ovarian tumour cells, *Br. J. Cancer*, 48, 515, 1983.

58. Lotzova, E., Savary, C., Freedman, R., and Bowen, J., Natural killer cell cytotoxic potential of patients with ovarian carcinoma and its modulation with virus-modified tumor cell extract, *Cancer Immunol. Immunother.*, 17, 124, 1984.

59. Lichtenstein, A., Berek, J., Bast, R., Spina, C., Hacker, N., Knapp, R., and Zighelboim, J., Activation of peritoneal lymphocyte cytotoxicity in patients with ovarian cancer by intraperitoneal treatment with Corynebacterium parvum, *J. Biol. Response Mod.*, 3, 371, 1984.

60. Lichtenstein, A., Berek, J., and Zighelboim, J., Natural killer inhibitory substance produced by the peritoneal cells of patients with ovarian cancer, *J. Natl. Cancer Inst.*, 74, 349, 1985.

61. Uchida, A. and Micksche, M., Natural killer cells in carcinomatous pleural effusions, *Cancer Immunother.*, 11, 131, 1981.

62. Onsrud, M., Adjuvant hydroxyprogesterone caproate in stage I endometrial carcinoma: changes in numbers and reactivities of some blood lymphocyte subpopulations, *Gynecol. Oncol.*, 14, 355, 1982.

63. Seltzer, V., Doyle, A., and Kadish, A., natural cytotoxicity in malignant and premalignant cervical neoplasia and enhancement of cytotoxicity with interferon, *Gynecol. Oncol.*, 15, 340, 1983.

64. Garam, T., Pulay, T., Bakacs, T., Svastits, E., Ringwald, G., Totpal, K., and Petranyi, G., NK and K cell activity in mammary carcinoma patients in relation to radiation therapy and the course of disease, in *NK Cells and Other Natural Effector Cells,* Herberman, R. B., Ed., Academic Press, New York, 1982, p 1189.

65. Pulay, T., Benczur, M., and Varga, M., Natural killer lymphocyte function in cervical cancer patients, *Neoplasma*, 29, 237, 1982.

66. Blomgren, H., Strender, L-E., Petrini, B., and Wasserman, J., Changes of the spontaneous cytotoxicity of the blood lymphocyte population following local radiation therapy for breast cancer, *Eur. J. Cancer Clin. Oncol.*, 18, 637, 1982.

67. Hovanessian, A., Youn, J., Buffet-Janvresse, C., Riviere, Y., Michelson, M., Lacour, J., and Lacour, F., Enhancement of natural killer cell activity and 2-5A synthetase in operable breast cancer patients treated with polyadenylic; polyuridylic. acid, *Cancer*, 55, 357, 1985.

68. Fulton, A., Heppner, G., Roi, L., Howard, L., Russo, J., and Brennan, M., Relationship of natural killer cell cytotoxicity to clinical and biomedical parameters of primary human breast cancer, *Breast Cancer Res. Treat.*, 4, 109, 1984.

69. Garner, W., Minton, J., James, A., and Hoffman, C., Suppressed natural killer cell surveillance in human breast cancer, *Surg. Forum,* 33, 422, 1982.

70. Garner, W., Minton, J., James, A., and Hoffmann, C., Human breast cancer and impaired NK cell function, *J. Surg. Oncol.*, 24, 64, 1983.

71. Hajto, T. and Lanzrein, C., Frequency of large granular lymphocytes in peripheral blood of healthy persons and breast cancer patients, *Cancer Immunol. Immunother.*, 16, 65, 1983.

72. Eremin, O., Coombs, R., and Ashby, J., Lymphocytes infiltrating human breast cancers lack K-cell activity and show low levels of NK-cell activity, *Br. J. Cancer*, 44, 166, 1981.

73. Heindenreich, W., Jagla, K., Schussler, J., Borner, P., Dehnhard, F., Kalden, J., Leibold, W., Peter, H., and Deicher, H., Spontaneous cell-mediated cytotoxicity (SCMC) and antibody-dependent cellular cytotoxicity (ADCC) in peripheral blood and draining lymph nodes of patients with mammary carcinoma, *Cancer Immunol. Immunother.*, 7, 65, 1979.

74. Uchida, A., Kolb, R., and Micksche, M., Generation of suppressor cells for natural killer activity in cancer patients after surgery, *J. Natl. Cancer Inst.*, 68, 735, 1982.

75. Mackay, I., Goodyear, M., Riglar, C., and Penschow, J., Effect on natural killer and antibody-dependent cellular cytotoxicity of adjuvant cytotoxic chemotherapy including melphalan in breast cancer, *Cancer Immunol. Immunother.*, 16, 98, 1983.

76. Cunningham-Rundles, S., Filippa, D., Braun, J. D., Antonelli, P., and Ashikari, H., Natural cytotoxicity of peripheral blood lymphocytes and regional lymph node cells in breast cancer in women, *J. Natl. Cancer Inst.,* 67, 585, 1981.

77. White, D., Jones, D., Cooke, T., and Kirkham, N., Natural killer (NK) activity in peripheral blood lymphocytes of patients with benign and malignant breast disease, *Br. J. Cancer,* 46, 611, 1982.

78. Steinhauer, E., Doyle, A., Reed, J., and Kadish, A., Natural killer cytotoxic factor induction by K562 cells in patients with advanced cancer: correlation with production of interferon, *J. Natl. Cancer Inst.,* submitted, 1985.

79. Forbes, J., Greco, F., and Oldham, R., Human natural cell-mediated cytotoxicity. II. Levels in neoplastic disease, *Cancer Immunol. Immunother.,* 11, 147, 1981.

80. Forbes, J., Greco, F., and Oldham, R., Natural cell-mediated cytotoxicity in human tumor patients, in *Natural Cell-Mediated Immunity Against Tumors,* Herberman, R. B., Ed., Academic Press, New York, 1980, p. 1031.

81. Moore, M. and Vose, B., Extravascular natural cytotoxicity in man: anti-K562 activity of lymph-node and tumour-infiltrating lyumphocytes, *Int. J. Cancer,* 27, 265, 1981.

82. Vose, B., Natural killers in human cancer: activity of tumor-infiltrating and draining lymph node lymphocytes, in *Natural Cell-Mediated Immunity against Tumors,* Herberman, R. B., Ed., Academic Press, New York, 1980, p 1081.

83. Liberati, A., Voelkel, J., Borden, E., Coates, A., Citrin, D., and Bryan, G., Influence of non-specific immunologic factors on prognosis in advanced bronchogenic carcinoma, *Cancer Immunol. Immunother.,* 13, 140, 1982.

84. Saijo, N., Shimizu, E., Irimajiri, N., Ozaki, A., Kimura, K., Takizawa, T., and Niitani, H., Analysis of natural killer activity and antibody-dependent cellular cytotoxicity in healthy volunteers and in patients with primary lung cancer and metastatic pulmonary tumors, *J. Cancer Res. Clin. Oncol.,* 102, 195, 1982.

85. Uchida, A. and Micksche, M., Suppressor cells for natural killer activity in carcinomatous pleural effusions of cancer patients, *Cancer Immunol. Immunother.,* 11, 255, 1981.

86. Saijo, N., Shimizu, E., Shibuya, M., Irimajiri, N., Takizawa, T., Eguchi, K., Shinki, T., Tominaga, K., Shimabukuru, Z., Taniguchi, T., and Hoshi, A., The effect of chemotherapy on natural killer activity and antibody dependent cell-mediated cytotoxicity in carcinoma of the lung, *Br. J. Cancer,* 46, 180, 1982.

87. Ito, M., Suzuki, H., Yamashita, N., Sugiyama, E., Maruyama, M., Sato, M., Iwata, M., and Yano, S., Beneficial effects of interleukin-2 on natural killer activity in lung cancer patients, *Anticancer Res.,* 4, 375, 1984.

88. Balch, C., Tilden, A., Dougherty, P., Cloud, G., and Abo, T., Heterogeneity of natural killer lymphocyte abnormalities in colon cancer patients, *Surgery,* 95, 63, 1984.

89. Waller, C., Gill, P., and MacLennan, I., Enhancement of lymphocyte-mediated cytotoxicity after tumor resection in patients with colorectal cancer, *J. Natl. Cancer Inst.,* 65, 223, 1980.

90. Vose, B., Gallagher, P., Moore, M., and Schofield, P., Specific and nonspecific lymphocyte cytotoxicity in colon carcinoma, *Br. J. Cancer,* 44, 846, 1981.

91. Griffith, C., Rees, R., Plats, A., Jermy, A., Peel, J., and Rogers, K., The nature of enhanced natural killer lymphocyte cytotoxicity during anesthesia and surgery in patients with benign disease and cancer, *Ann. Surg.,* 200, 753, 1984.

92. Lang, I., Feuer, L., Nekam, K., Szigeti, A., Gergely, P., and Petranyi, G., Glutaurine enhances the depressed NK cell activity of tumor patients, *Immunol. Commun.,* 12, 519, 1983.

93. Tanaka, N., Hashimoto, T., Matsui, T., Ohida, J., Ono, M., and Orita, K., Natural cytotoxic reactivity of peripheral blood lymphocytes from digestive tract cancer patients against a colon cancer cell line and virus-infected hela cells, *Gann,* 74, 419, 1983.

94. Son, K., Kew, M., and Rabson, A., Depressed natural killer cell activity in patients with hepatocellular carcinoma, *Cancer,* 50, 2820, 1982.

95. Funa, K., Nilsson, B., Jacobsson, G., and Alm, G., Decreased natural killer cell activity and interferon production by leucocytes in patients with adenocarcinoma of the pancreas, *Br. J. Cancer,* 50, 231, 1984.

96. Funa, K., Alm, G., Ronnblom, L., and Oberg, K., Evaluation of the natural killer cell — interferon system in patients with mid-gut carcinoid tumours treated with leucocyte interferon, *Clin. Exp. Immunol.,* 53, 716, 1983.

97. Vilien, M., Wolf, H., and Rasmussen, F., Titration of natural and disease-related cytotoxicity of lymphocytes from bladder cancer patients, *Cancer Immunol. Immunother.,* 8, 189, 1980.

98. Ratliff, T., McCool, R., and Catalona, W., Antibody-dependent and spontaneous lympholysis in urologic cancer patients, *Br. J. Cancer,* 39, 667, 1979.

99. Wirth, M., Schmitz-Drager, B., and Ackermann, R., Functional properties of natural killer cells in carcinoma of the prostate, *J. Urol.,* 133, 973, 1985.

100. Okabe, T., Ackermann, R., Wirth, M., and Frohmuller, H., Cell-mediated cytotoxicity in patients with cancer of the prostate, *J. Urol.,* 122, 628, 1979.
101. Kalland, T. and Haukaas, S., Effect of treatment with diethylstilbestrol-polyestradiol phosphate or estramustine phosphate (Estracyt) on natural killer cell activity in patients with prostatic cancer, *Invest. Urol.,* 18, 437, 1981.
102. Gerson, J. and Herberman, R., Systemic and in situ natural killer activity in patients with neuroblastoma, *Prog. Cancer Res. Ther.,* 12, 344, 1980.
103. Braun, D., Penn, R., and Harris, J., Regulation of natural killer cell function by glass-adherent cells in patients with primary intracranial malignancies, *Neurosurgery,* 15, 29, 1984.
104. Einhorn, S., Ahre, A., Blomgren, H., Johansson, B., Mellstedt, H., and Strander, H., Interferon and natural killer activity in multiple myeloma. Lack of correlation between interferon-induced enhancement of natural killer activity and clinical response to human interferon-a, *Int. J. Cancer,* 30, 167, 1982.
105. Hawrylowicz, C., Rees, R., Hancock, B., and Potter, C., Depressed spontaneous natural killing and interferon augmentation in patients with malignant lymphoma, *Eur. J. Cancer Clin. Oncol.,* 18, 1081, 1982.
106. Rotstein, S., Baral, E., Blomgren, H., and Johansson, B., In vitro radiosensitivity of the spontaneous cytotoxicity of blood lymphocytes in patients with untreated Hodgkin's disease, *Eur. J. Cancer Clin. Oncol.,* 19, 1405, 1983.
107. Ruco, L., Procopio, A., Uccini, S., Marcorelli, E., and Baroni, C., Natural killer activity in spleens and lymph nodes from patients with Hodgkin's disease, *Cancer Res.,* 42, 2063, 1982.
108. Levy, S., Tempe, J., Aleksijevic, A., Giron, C., Oberling, F., Mayer, S., and Lang, J., Depressed NK cell activity of peripheral blood mononuclear cells in untreated Hodgkin's disease: enhancing effect of interferon in vitro, *Scand. J. Haematol.,* 33, 386, 1984.
109. Al Sam, S., Jones, D., Payne, S., and Wright, D., Natural killer (NK) activity in the spleen of patients with Hodgkin's disease and controls, *Br. J. Cancer,* 46, 806, 1982.
110. Gupta, S. and Fernandes, G., Spontaneous and antibody-dependent cellular cytotoxicity by lymphocyte subpopulations in peripheral blood and spleen from adult untreated patients with Hodgkin's disease, *Clin. Exp. Immunol.,* 45, 205, 1981.
111. Gupta, S. and Fernandes, G., Natural killing in patients with Hodgkin's Disease, in *NK Cells and Other Natural Effector Cells,* Herberman, R. B., Ed., Academic Press, New York, 1982, p 1201.
112. Cortesina, C., Sartoris, A., Di Fortunato, V., Cavallo, G., Morra, B., Bussi, M., Beatrice, F., Poggio, E., Marcato, P., and Rendine, S., Natural killer-mediated cytotoxicity in patients with laryngeal carcinoma, *Ann. Otol. Rhinol. Laryngol.,* 93, 189, 1984.
113. Gu, S., Petrini, B., Stedingk, L. V., Thyresson, N., and Wasserman, J., Blood lymphocyte subpopulations in mycosis fungoides and their functions in vitro, *Acta. Dermatol. Venereol.,* 61, 487, 1981.
114. Jensen, J., Thestrup-Pedersen, K., Ahrons, S., and Zachariae, H., The immunological profile of mycosis fungoides, *Clin. Exp. Immunol.,* 50, 397, 1982.
115. Levy, S., Tempe, J., Caussade, P., Aleksijevic, A., Grosshans, E., Mayer, S., and Lang, J., Stage-related decrease in natural killer cell activity in untreated patients with mycosis fungoides, *Cancer Immunol. Immunother.,* 18, 138, 1984.
116. Neilan, B., Vonderheid, E., and O'Neill, K., Natural cell-mediated cytotoxicity in cutaneous T-cell lymphomas, *J. Invest. Dermatol.,* 81, 176, 1983.
117. Laroche, L. and Kaiserlian, D., Decreased natural killer cell activity in cutaneous T-cell lymphomas, *N. Engl. J. Med.,* 308, 101, 1983.
118. Herberman, R., Interferon and cytotoxic effector cells, in *Interferon,* Vilcek, J. and De Maeyer, E., Eds., Elsevier Sience, Amsterdam, 1984, 61.
119. Herberman, R. B., Immunoregulation and natural killer cells, *Mol. Immunol.,* 19, 1313, 1982.
120. Kimber, I. and Moore, M., Mechanism and regulation of natural cytotoxicity, *Exp. Cell Biol.,* 53, 69, 1985.
121. Roder, J. C., Karre, K., and Kiessling, R., Natural killer cells, *Prog. Allergy,* 28, 66, 1981.
122. Fernandes, G. and Gupta, S., Natural killing and antibody-dependent cytotoxicity by lymphocyte subpopulations in young and aging humans, *J. Clin. Immunol.,* 1, 141, 1981.
123. Thompson, J., Wekstein, D., Rhoades, J., Kirkpatrick, C., Brown, S., Roszman, T., Straus, R., and Tietz, N., The immune status of healthy centenarians, *J. Am. Geriatr. Soc.,* 32, 274, 1984.
124. Onsrud, M., Age dependent changes in some human lymphocyte subpopulations. Changes in natural killer cell activity, *Acta Pathol. Microbiol. Scand., Sec. C,* 89, 55, 1981.
125. Bash, J. and Vogel, D., Cellular immunosenescence in F344 rats: decreased natural killer (NK) cell activity involves changes in regulatory interactions between NK cells, interferon, prostaglandin and macrophages, *Mech. Ageing Dev.,* 24, 49, 1984.
126. Golub, S., Niitsuma, M., Kawate, N., Cochran, A., and Holmes, E., NK activity of tumor infiltrating and lymph node lymphocytes in human pulmonary tumors, in *NK Cells and Other Natural Effector Cells,* Herberman, R. B., Ed., Academic Press, New York, 1982, p 1113.

127. Eremin, O., NK cell activity in the blood, tumour-draining lymph nodes and primary tumours of women with mammary carcinoma, in *Natural Cell-Mediated Immunity against Tumors,* Herberman, R. B., Ed., Academic Press, New York, 1980, p 1011.

128. Kimber, I., Moore, M., Howell, A., and Wilkinson, M., Native and inducible levels of natural cytotoxicity in lymph nodes draining mammary carcinoma, *Cancer Immunol. Immunother.,* 15, 32, 1983.

129. Vose, B., Vanky, F., Argov, S., and Klein, E., Natural cytotoxicity in man: activity of lymph node and tumor infiltrating lymphocytes, *Eur. J. Immunol.,* 7, 753, 1977.

130. Hutchinson, G. H., Symes, M. O., and Williamson, R. C. N., Cytotoxicity of lymphocytes from blood, tumor and regional lymph nodes against K562 cells and autoplastic colorectal tumor cells, *Br. J. Cancer,* 46, 682, 1982.

131. Mantovani, A., Allavena, P., Sessa, C., Bolis, G., and Mangioni, C., Natural killer activity of lymphoid cells isolated from human ascitic ovarian tumors, *Int. J. Cancer,* 25, 573, 1980.

132. Moore, K. and Moore, J., Systemic and in-situ natural killer activity in tumour-bearing rats, *Br. J. Cancer,* 39, 636, 1979.

133. Niitsuma, M., Golub, S., Edelstein, R., and Holmes, E., Lymphoid cells infiltrating human pulmonary tumors: effect of intralesional BCG injection, *J. Natl. Cancer Inst.,* 67, 997, 1981.

134. Moy, P., Holmes, E., and Golub, S., Depression of natural killer cytotoxic activity in lymphocytes infiltrating human pulmonary tumors, *Cancer Res.,* 45, 57, 1985.

135. Uchida, A. and Micksche, M., Lysis of fresh human tumor cells by autologous large granular lymphocytes from peripheral blood and pleural effusions, *Int. J. Cancer,* 32, 37, 1983.

136. Balch, C., Tilden, A., Dougherty, P., and Cloud, G., Depressed levels of granular lymphocytes with natural killer (NK) cell function in 247 cancer patients, *Ann. Surg.,* 198, 192, 1983.

137. Hellstrom, K. E., Hellstrom, I., Nelson, K., Forstom, J. W., and Nepom, G. T., Suppressor factors in tumor immunity, *Transplant. Proc.,* 16, 470, 1984.

138. Peter, H. H., Pavie-Fischer, J., Fridman, W. H., Aubert, C., Cesarini, J. P., Roubin, R., and Kourilsky, F. M., Cell-mediated cytotoxicity in vitro of human lymphocytes against a tissue culture melanoma cell line (IGR3), *J. Immunol.,* 115, 539, 1975.

139. Merrill, J. E., Ullberg, M., and Jondal, M., Influence of IgG and IgM receptor triggering on human natural killer cell cytotoxicity measured on the level of the single effector cell, *Eur. J. Immunol.,* 11, 536, 1981.

140. Perussia, B., Trinchieri, G., and Cerottini, J. C., Functional studies of Fc receptor-bearing human lymphocytes: effect of treatment with proteolytic enzymes, *J. Immunol.,* 123, 681, 1979.

141. Pape, G. R., Troye, M., Axelsson, B., and Perlmann, P., Simultaneous occurrence of immunoglobulin-dependent and immunoglobulin-independent mechanisms in natural cytotoxicity of human lymphocytes, *J. Immunol.,* 122, 2251, 1979.

142. Kay, H. D., Bonnard, G. D., and Herberman, R. B., Evaluation of the role of IgG antibodies in human natural cell-mediated cytotoxicity against the myeloid cell line K562, *J. Immunol.,* 122, 675, 1979.

143. Dorval, G. and Pross, H. F., Immune complexes in cancer, in *Immune Complexes: Their Significance in Clinical Medicine,* L. R. Spinoza, Ed., Futura Publishing, Miami, Fla., 1983, p 161.

144. Roder, J. C., Rosen, A., Fenyo, E. M., and Troy, F. A., Target-effector interaction in the natural killer cell system: isolation of target structures, *Proc. Natl. Acad. Sci.,* 76, 1405, 1979.

145. Zaunders, J., Werkmeister, J., McCarthy, W. H., and Hersey, P., Characterization of antigens recognized by natural killer cells in cell-culture supernatants, *Br. J. Cancer,* 43, 5, 1981.

146. Blazar, B. A., Fitzgerald, J., Sutton, L., and Strome, M., Increased sensitivity to natural killing in Raji cells is due to effector recognition of molecules appearing on target cell membranes following EBV cycle induction, *Clin. Exp. Immunol.,* 54, 31, 1983.

147. Bishop, G., Glorioso, J., and Schwartz, S., Relationship between expression of herpes simplex virus glycoproteins and susceptibility of target cells to human natural killer activity, *J. Exp. Med.,* 157, 1544, 1983.

148. Yogeeswaran, G., Gronberg, A., Hansson, M., Dalianis, T., Kiessling, R., and Welsh, R. M., Correlation of glycosphingolipids and sialic acid in Yac-1 lymphoma variants with their sensitivity to natural killer-cell-mediated lysis, *Int. J. Cancer,* 28, 517, 1981.

149. Young, W. W., Durdik, J. M., Urdal, D., Hakomori, S. I., and Henney, C. S., Glycolipid expression in lymphoma cell variants: chemical quantity, immunologic reactivity, and correlations with susceptibility to NK cells, *J. Immunol.,* 126, 1, 1981.

150. Durdik, J. M., Beck, B., Clark, E., and Henney, C., Characterization of a lymphoma cell variant selectively resistant to natural killer cells, *J. Immunol.,* 125, 683, 1980.

151. Harris, J., Chin, J., Jewett, M., Kennedy, M., and Gorczynski, R., Monoclonal antibodies against SSEA-1 antigen: binding properties and inhibition of human natural killer cell activity against target cells bearing SSEA-1 antigen, *J. Immunol.,* 132, 2502, 1984.

152. Werkmeister, J., Pross, H. P., and Roder, J. C., Modulation of K562 cells with sodium butyrate. Association of impaired NK susceptibility with sialic acid and analysis of other parameters, *Int. J. Cancer*, 32, 71, 1983.

153. Forbes, J. T., Bretthauer, R. K., and Oeltmann, T. N., Mannose 6-fructose 1- and fructose 6-phosphates inhibit human natural killer cell-mediated cytotoxicity, *Proc. Natl. Acad. Sci. U.S.A.*, 78, 5797, 1981.

154. Werkmeister, J., Roder, J., Curry, C., and Pross, H., The effect of unphosphorylated and phosphorylated sugar moieties on human and mouse natural killer cell activity. Is there selective inhibition at the level of target recognition and lytic acceptor site?, *Cell. Immunol.*, 80, 172, 1983.

155. Ortaldo, J., Timonen, T., and Herberman, R., Inhibition of activity of human NK and K cells by simple sugars: discrimination between binding and postbinding events, *Clin. Immunol. Immunopathol.*, 31, 439, 1984.

156. Ades, E. W., Hinson, A., and Decker, J. M., Effector cell sensitivity to sugar moieties. I. Inhibition of human natural killer cell activity by monosaccharides, *Immunobiology*, 160, 248, 1981.

157. Stutman, O., Dien, P., Wisun, R. E., and Lattime, E. C., Natural cytotoxic cells against solid tumors in mice: blocking of cytotoxicity by D-mannose, *Proc. Natl. Acad. Sci. U.S.A.*, 77, 2895, 1980.

158. Berek, J., Bast, R. J., Lichtenstein, A., Hacker, N., Spina, C., Lagasse, L., Knapp, R., and Zighelboim, J., Lymphocyte cytotoxicity in the peritoneal cavity and blood of patients with ovarian cancer, *Obstet. Gynecol.*, 64, 708, 1984.

159. Onsrud, M., Serum-mediated immunosuppression: a possible tumor marker in patients with ovarian carcinoma, *Gynecol. Oncol.*, 21, 94, 1985.

160. Saxena, R., Saxena, Q., and Adler, W., Mechanism of loss of natural killer activity in P815 ascites tumor bearing DBA/2 mice, *Natl. Immunol. Cell Growth Regul.*, 3, 34, 1983.

161. Zighelboim, J., Lichtenstein, A., Bick, A., and Mickel, R., Inhibition of natural killer cell activity by a soluble substance released by rat peritoneal cells, *Cancer Res.*, 43, 1984, 1983.

162. Lichtenstein, A., Mickel, R., and Zighelboim, J., Inhibition of natural killer cell lysis by natural killer-inhibitory substance: mechanism of suppression, *Cell. Immunol.*, 80, 66, 1983.

163. Zoller, M. and Matzku, S., Rat macrophages inhibit natural killer (NK) cell activity against adherent growing target cells, *Immunobiology*, 163, 497, 1982.

164. Goodwin, J. and Williams, R., Suppressor cells — a recent conceptual epidemic, *J. Clin. Lab. Immunol.*, 2, 89, 1979.

165. Waldmann, T. A., Broder, S., Blaese, R. M., Durm, M., Goldman, C., and Muul, L., Role of suppressor cells in human disease, in *Biological Basis of Immunodeficiency*, Gelfand, E. W. and Dosch, H. M., Eds., Raven Press, New York, 1980, p. 223.

166. Zoller, M. and Wigzell, H., Normally occurring inhibitory cells for natural killer cell activity. II. Characterization of the inhibitory cell, *Cell. Immunol.*, 74, 27, 1982.

167. Lotzova, E., C. Parvum-mediated suppression of the phenomenon of natural killing and its analysis, in *Natural Cell-Mediated Immunity Against Tumours*, Herbermann, R. B., Ed., Academic Press, New York, 1980, p. 735.

168. Tarkkanen, J., Saksela, E., and Paavolainen, M., Suppressor cells of natural killer activity in normal and tumor-bearing individuals, *Clin. Immunol. Immunopath.*, 28, 29, 1983.

169. D'Amore, P. J. and Golub, S., Suppression of human NK cell cytotoxicity by an MLC-generated cell population, *J. Immunol.*, 134, 272, 1985.

170. Ullberg, M., Merrill, J., and Jondal, M., Interferon-induced NK augmentation in humans. An analysis of target recognition, effector cell recruitment and effector cell recycling, *Scand. J. Immunol.*, 14, 285, 1981.

171. Rubin, P., Pross, H. F., and Roder, J. C., Studies of human natural killer cells. II. Analysis at the single cell level, *J. Immunol.*, 128, 2553, 1982.

172. Saksela, E., Timonen, T., and Cantell, K., Human natural killer cell activity is augmented by interferon via recruitment of "pre-NK" cells, *Scand. J. Immunol.*, 10, 257, 1979.

173. Targan, S., and Dorey, F., Interferon activation of 'pre-spontaneous killer' (pre-SK) cells and alteration in kinetics of lysis of both 'pre-SK' and active SK cells, *J. Immunol.*, 124, 2157, 1980.

174. Herberman, R. B., Djeu, J. Y., Ortaldo, J. R., Holden, H., West, W., and Bonnard, G. D., Role of interferon in augmentation of natural and antibody-dependent cell-mediated cytotoxicity, *Cancer Treat. Rep.*, 62, 1893, 1978.

175. Brunda, M., Taramelli, D., Holden, H., and Varesio, L., Suppression of in vitro maintenance and interferon-mediated augmentation of natural killer cell activity by adherent peritoneal cells from normal mice, *J. Immunol.*, 130, 1974, 1983.

176. Trinchieri, G., Santoli, D., Granato, D., and Perussia, B., Antagonistic effects of interferons on the cytotoxicity mediated by natural killer cells, *Fed. Proc.*, 40, 2705, 1981.

177. Saito, T., Ruffmann, R., Welker, R. D., Herberman, R. B., and Chirigos, M. A., Development of hyporesponsiveness of natural killer cells to augmentation of activity after multiple treatments with biological response modifiers, *Cancer Immunol. Immunother.*, 19, 130, 1985.

178. Steinhauer, E., Doyle, A., and Kadish, A., Human natural killer cytotoxic factor (NKCF): role of IFN-gamma[1], *J. Immunol.*, in press, 1985.

179. Wright, S. and Bonavida, B., Selective lysis of NK-sensitive target cells by a soluble mediator released from murine spleen cells and human peripheral blood lymphocytes, *J. Immunol.*, 126, 1516, 1981.

180. Herberman, R., Allavena, P., Scala, G., Djeu, J., Kasahara, T., Domzig, W., Procopio, A., Blanca, I., Ortaldo, J., and Oppenheim, J., Cytokine production by human large granular lymphocytes (LGL), in *Proc. Inter. Symp. Natural Killer Activity Reg.*, Kyoto, Japan, Excerpta Medica, Amsterdam, 1983 p. 409.

181. Herberman, R., Multiple functions of natural killer cells, including immunoregulation as well as resistance to tumor growth, *Concepts Immunopathol.*, 1, 96, 1985.

182. Henney, C., Kuribayashi, K., Kern, D., and Gillis, S., Interleukin-2 augments natural killer cell activity, *Nature (London)*, 291, 335, 1981.

183. London, L., Perussia, B., and Trinchieri, G., Induction of proliferation in vitro of resting human natural killer cells: expression of surface activation antigens, *J. Immunol.*, 134, 718, 1985.

184. Van De Griend, R. J., Van Krimpen, B. A., Roteltap, C. P. H., and Bolhuis, R. L. H., Rapidly expanded activated human killer cell clones have strong anti-tumor cell activity and have the surface phenotype of either T gamma, T non-gamma or null cells, *J. Immunol.*, 132, 3185, 1984.

185. Suzuki, R., Handa, K., Itoh, K., and Kumagai, K., Natural killer (NK) cells as a responder to interleukin 2 (IL2). I. Proliferative response and establishment of cloned cells, *J. Immunol.*, 130, 981, 1983.

186. Robb, R., Interleukin 2: the molecule and its function, *Immunol. Today*, 5, 203, 1984.

187. Ruscetti, F., Biology of interleukin-2, *Surv. Immunol. Res.*, 3, 122, 1984.

188. Ravikumar, T., Rodrick, M., Steele, G., Marrazo, J., O'Dwyer, P., Dodson, T., and King, V., Interleukin generation in experimental colon cancer of rats: effects of tumor growth and tumor therapy, *J. Natl. Cancer Inst.*, 74, 893, 1985.

189. Moller-Larsen, F., Moller-Larsen, A., and Haahr, S., The influence of general anesthesia and surgery on cell-mediated cytotoxicity and interferon production, *J. Clin. Lab. Immunol.*, 12, 69, 1983.

190. Ryhanen, P., Huttunen, K., and Ilonen, J., Natural killer cell activity after open-heart surgery, *Acta Anaesthesiol. Scand.*, 28, 490, 1984.

191. Schantz, S. P., Romsdahl, M. M., Babcock, G. F., Nishioka, K., and Goepfert, H., The effect of surgery on natural killer cell activity in head and neck cancer patients: in vitro reversal of a postoperatively suppressed immunosurveillance system, *Laryngoscope*, 95, 588, 1985.

192. Kedar, E., Katz-Gross, A., Chriqui-Zeira, E., and Bercowitz, H., Suppression by tumor growth of T cell growth factor production in mouse lymphoid cell cultures, *J. Biol. Response Mod.*, 3, 547, 1984.

193. Burger, C., Elgert, K., and Farrar, W., Interleukin 2 (IL-2) activity during tumor growth: IL-2 production kinetics, absorption of and responses to exogenous IL-2, *Cell. Immunol.*, 84, 228, 1984.

194. Elliott, L., Brooks, W., and Roszman, T., Cytokinetic basis for the impaired activation of lymphocytes from patients with primary intracranial tumors, *J. Immunol.*, 132, 1208, 1984.

195. Fontana, A., Hengartner, H., De Tribolet, N., and Weber, E., Glioblastoma cells release interleukin 1 and factors inhibiting interleukin 2-mediated effects, *J. Immunol.*, 132, 1837, 1984.

196. Hersey, P., Bindon, C., Czerniecki, M., Spurling, A., Wass, J., and McCarthy, W., Inhibition of interleukin 2 production by factors released from tumor cells, *J. Immunol.*, 131, 2837, 1983.

197. Koch, B., Regnat, W., Solbach, W., Lanz, R., Hermanek, P., and Kalden, J. R., Inteleukin-2 production in peripheral blood mononuclear cells of patients with gastrointestinal tumors, *J. Clin. Lab. Immunol.*, 13, 171, 1984.

198. Herman, J., Kew, M., and Rabson, A., Defective interleukin-1 production by monocytes from patients with malignant disease. Interferon increases IL-1 production, *Cancer Immunol. Immunother.*, 16, 182, 1984.

199. Pollack, S., Micali, A., Kinne, D. W., Enker, W. E., Geller, N., Oettgen, H. F., and Hoffman, M. K., Endotoxin-induced in vitro release of interleukin-1 by cancer patients' monocytes: relation to stage of disease, *Int. J. Cancer*, 32, 733, 1983.

200. Keong, A., Herman, J., and Rabson, A., Supernatant derived from a human hepatocellular carcinoma cell line (PLC/PRF/5) depresses natural killer (NK) cell activity, *Cancer Immunol. Immunother.*, 15, 183, 1983.

201. Sundar, S., Bergeron, J., and Menezes, J., Purified plasminogen activating factor produced by malignant lymphoid cells abrogates lymphocyte cytotoxicity, *Clin. Exp. Immunol.*, 56, 701, 1984.

202. Koren, H. and Leung, K., Modulation of human NK cells by interferon and prostaglandin E2, *Mol. Immunol.*, 19, 1341, 1982.

203. Hall, T. and Brostoff, J., Inhibition of human natural killer cell activity by prostaglandin D2, *Immunol. Lett.*, 7, 141, 1983.

204. Hall, T., Chen, S., Brostoff, J., and Lydyard, P., Modulation of human natural killer cell activity by pharmacological mediators, *Clin. Exp. Immunol.*, 54, 493, 1983.

205. Bankhurst, A., The modulation of human natural killer cell activity by prostaglandins, *J. Clin. Lab. Immunol.,* 7, 85, 1982.

206. Brunda, M. J., Herberman, R., and Holden, H., Inhibition of murine natural killer cell activity by prostaglandins, *J. Immunol.,* 124, 2682, 1980.

207. Droller, M., Schneider, M., and Perlmann, P., A possible role of prostaglandins in the inhibition of natural and antibody-dependent cell-mediated cytotoxicity against tumor cells, *Cell. Immunol.,* 39, 165, 1978.

208. Ching, C., Ching, N., Seto, D., and Hokama, Y., Relationships of prostaglandin levels and natural killer (NK) cell cytotoxicity of mononuclear cells in cord blood, *J. Med.,* 15, 233, 1984.

209. Zielinski, C., Gisinger, C., Binder, C., Mannhalter, J., and Eibl, M., Regulation of NK cell activity by prostaglandic E_2: the role of T cells, *Cell. Immunol.,* 87, 65, 1984.

210. Herman, J. and Rabson, A., Prostaglandin E2 depresses natural cytotoxicity by inhibiting interleukin-1 production by large granular lymphocytes, *Clin. Exp. Immunol.,* 57, 380, 1984.

211. Rola-Pleszczynski, M., Gagnon, L., and Sirois, P., Natural cytotoxic cell activity enhanced by leukotriene B4: Modulation by cyclooxygenase and lipoxygenase inhibitors, in *Icosanoids and Cancer,* Thaler-Dao, H., dePaulet, A. C., and Paoletti, R., Eds., Raven Press, New York, 1984, p 235.

212. Gisinger, C., Zielinski, C., and Eibl, M. M., Relevance of cellular interactions in PGE_2-mediated natural killer cell inhibition, in *Icosanoids and Cancer,* Thaler-Dao, H., dePaulet, A. C., and Paoletti, R., Eds., Raven Press, New York, 1984 p 279.

213. Kay, N. and Zarling, J., Imparied natural killer activity in patients with chronic lymphocytic leukemia is associated with a deficiency of azurophilic cytoplasmic granules in putative NK cells, *Blood,* 63, 305, 1984.

214. Uchida, A., Colot, M., and Micksche, M., Suppression of natural killer cell activity by adherent effusion cells of cancer patients. Suppression of motility, binding capacity and letal hit of NK cells, *Br. J. Cancer,* 49, 17, 1984.

215. Badger, A. M., Oh, S. K., and Moolten, F. R., Differential effects of an immunosuppressive fraction from ascites fluid of patients with ovarian cancer on spontaneous and antibody-dependent cytotoxicity, *Cancer Res.,* 41, 1133, 1981.

216. Hersey, P., Edwards, A., Milton, G. W., and McCarthy, W. H., No evidence for an association between natural killer cell activity and prognosis in melanoma patients, *Natl. Immun. Cell Growth Regul.,* 3, 87, 1984.

217. Pross, H. F. and Baines, M. C., Unpublished observation.

Chapter 5

ALTERATIONS IN MACROPHAGE FUNCTION IN TUMOR-BEARING HOSTS

D.S. Nelson

TABLE OF CONTENTS

I. INTRODUCTION

There has long been an interest in the idea that macrophages might be involved in resistance to cancer.[1] Since the discovery that activated macrophages could recognize and selectively destroy tumor cells in vitro[2,3] the idea has become more attractive. Evidence has been sought and found that macrophages may restrict the growth of primary tumors, the formation of metastases, and the emergence of tumor cells from the dormant state. The restriction of tumor growth and spread by macrophages requires that they be available and adequate in number and function, including mobility, to restrict either the dissemination of cells from a primary tumor or their establishment and multiplication at metastatic sites. This in turn implies that the host must possess effective mechanisms to deliver and activate macrophages. As with so many aspects of tumor biology, the results of numerous studies are sometimes conflicting and confusing, and now include evidence that macrophages can sometimes stimulate tumor cells. The complex relationships between tumor and host not only vary with the tumor and the host, but can also change with time during the growth of one tumor. Behind any discussion of tumor-macrophage interactions there lies the fact of macrophage heterogeneity: not only is there diversity between and within populations, but the activation of populations and individual cells can change quite dramatically with time. It is the purpose of this chapter to examine macrophage function during tumor growth, especially in well-studied experimental systems, the ways in which changes in function are brought about, and the significance both for host-tumor relationships and host immunity generally.

II. ANTITUMOR MONOCYTES AND MACROPHAGES

A. Occurrence

The central questions here are whether tumor-bearing shots possess mononuclear phagocytes with antitumor activity, whether these cells can be delivered to sites of tumor growth, and whether they can act effectively after delivery. An important question underlying these is whether monocytes and macrophages of normal animals (including man) have antitumor activity, the effectiveness of which may determine whether or not primary or transplanted tumors emerge and grow. This question is somewhat peripheral to the present discussion and has been discussed in detail by others,[4-6] but requires some comment.

The ability of human peripheral blood monocytes to damage cultured tumor cells has been extensively reported. Assays have included the measurement of rapid cytolysis by means of ^{51}Cr release,[7] slower cytotoxicity by means of ^{3}H-thymidine or ^{125}I-iododeoxyuridine release after prolonged (48 to 72 hr) incubation,[8] and cytostasis by means of ^{3}H-thymidine uptake.[9] Targets have included a variety of lymphoid and myeloid tumor cell lines, such as the erythromyeloid leukemia K562,[7,10] human ovarian and other cancer cells,[8,9] other human cancer cell lines,[11,12] transformed fibroblasts,[12,13] and actinomycin D-treated human and mouse tumor cells.[14]

There are, however, some reservations about the interpretation of these studies. NK cells may contaminate freshly isolated monocyte preparations, but be lost when adherent cell cultures are washed after 24 hr or more.[15] Prolonged culture and washing of human blood monocytes may also lead to loss of their spontaneous cytotoxicity, which can be recovered or induced by stimulation with bacterial lipopolysaccharide (LPS), or preparations containing lymphokines.[15-17] Monoclonal antibodies to NK cells have also been used to deplete monocytes of NK cells, with a reduction in cytotoxicity in one study,[15] but an increase (against a mouse tumor cell line) in another.[18]

Despite these reservations it is worth noting that spontaneous "monocyte-mediated" cytotoxicity or cytostasis in cancer patients has been reported to be normal,[12] slightly impaired,[9] impaired according to the extent of disease (lung cancer[19]), or with nontumor targets and prolonged preincubation, markedly impaired.[20] Impairment of the LPS-inducible cytotoxic activity of monocyte-derived macrophages has also been reported in patients with head and neck, breast and gynecological cancers, but not colon or some hematological cancers.[21,22]

Blood monocytes can also effect antibody-dependent cell-mediated cytotoxicity (ADCC). With nontumor targets this capacity has been reported to be impaired in patients with Hodgkin's disease.[23] In another study, no impairment was found in patients with Hodgkin's or non-Hodgkin's lymphoma, lung or breast cancer, very slight impairment in patients with melanoma or gastrointestinal cancer, and stimulation in a group of patients with gastrointestinal cancer of limited extent.[24]

Macrophages from other sites in man are rather less readily studied, as procedures to obtain them may not be justified in the absence of disease. Nevertheless (and with reservations similar to those above) spontaneous cytotoxicity has been observed with macrophages from cantharidin blisters,[11] milk (early lactation) and from the peritoneal cavities of women undergoing surgery for nonmalignant gynecological conditions.[25] Alveolar macrophages from subjects without lung disease have been reported to be cytotoxic to long-term human tumor cell lines,[26] not cytotoxic to transformed mouse kidney cells,[27] or not cytotoxic to freshly explanted lung cancer and melanoma lines.[28] In contrast, alveolar macrophages from patients with lung cancer were cytotoxic to those same freshly explanted targets[28] and, in other studies, cytotoxic or cytostatic to lung cancer cell lines.[19,26] Blister macrophages from cancer patients were cytotoxic to two human cancer cell lines.[11]

The most commonly studied macrophages in experimental animals are peritoneal macrophages in mice and rats. There is general agreement that resident peritoneal macrophages from microbiologically clean mice are not cytotoxic to tumor cells.[29-31] Similarly, resident alveolar macrophages have also been found to be inactive.[32] It is less clear whether the cytotoxic activity sometimes found among resident peritoneal cells of rats is a normal activity or is a consequence of low grade infection, which appears to be more common among rat than mouse colonies.[6,33,34] Cytotoxicity of resident peritoneal macrophages from germ-free rats has been described, but was restricted to tumors with viral antigens.[35] Macrophages in inflammatory peritoneal exudates induced in mice by agents that do not activate macrophages are generally not cytotoxic, unless the eliciting agent contains LPS.[29,36-38] Again, the situation with rats is less clear.[6,33,39] A useful analysis of the cytokinetics of macrophage-mediated cytotoxicity has been made by Normann and Cornelius.[40]

The carriage of tumors that induce concomitant immunity led to the development of cytotoxic macrophages in the peritoneal cavities of mice. These cells were detectable by means of assays involving slow (48 hr) release of ^{3}H-thymidine or ^{125}I-iododeoxyuridine, but not assays of rapid ^{51}Cr release.[37] Cytotoxic macrophages may also be present in mice,[41,42] rats,[33,43] and hamsters[44] with concomitant immunity to other tumors. Somewhat different from concomitant immunity is the tumor dormant state, in which microscopic deposits of tumor cells persist, generally undetected, after primary treatment.[45,46] This is clearly of great clinical importance. Experimental models exist, and in one well-studied model — L5178Y lymphoma in DBA/2 mice — cytotoxic macrophages appear to be the effector cells maintaining the dormant state.[47]

The activity of tumor-associated macrophages is of great interest and is considered in detail in relation to metastasis by Haskill elsewhere in this volume. Suffice it to say here that growing tumors in man and experimental animals generally contain macrophages and that in some cases the macrophages have been found to possess antitumor activity, including a capacity for ADCC.[9,48-50] Despite initial hopes[51] it has proved difficult to relate the growth rate or metastatic capacity of tumors to their content of macrophages, either in experimental animals[52-54] or in man.[55] In one recent study of mouse mammary tumors, macrophages from metastatic tumors were more commonly cytotoxic in vitro than those from nonmetastasizing tumors.[56] The pattern of macrophage distribution and function also differed between metastasizing and nonmetastasizing tumors.[57] Macrophage depletion has sometimes been found to potentiate the growth of transplanted syngeneic tumors[58] but this has not been a generally observed phenomenon.[52] Some of our own studies involved three transplanted tumors in DA rats: a methylcholanthrene-induced fibrosarcoma (D8) a metastatic variant of that tumor (D8M) and a metastasizing spontaneous adenocarcinoma (ST2). All had been passaged at least twice. After depletion of macrophages, D8 grew faster in the feet of recipient rats. D8M grew less well and ST2 not only grew poorly but failed to metastasize.[59] It seems that tumors differ from each other in the nature of their relationship with infiltrating host macrophages. Some of the apparent discrepancies may be related to the ability of some macrophages to stimulate tumor cells, even if they have at one stage in their lives been cytotoxic (see Section III.). One of the curious features of tumor-associated macrophages in mice is their very high rate of proliferation.[60,61]

Macrophages in lymph nodes draining the sites of tumor growth have also been of interest. Sinus histiocytosis — a marked increase in the number of macrophages lining lymphoid sinuses — was thought to be an indicator of a good prognosis in breast and other human cancers.[62,63] More recently, this change has been linked to more aggressive growth.[64] Again, the diversity of individual tumor-macrophage relationships may preclude simple generalization.

B. Mechanisms of Stimulation and Delivery of Macrophages

It seems probable that the mechanism operating most commonly throughout life to activate macrophages is that of delayed-type hypersensitivity (DTH).[65] In the expression of DTH a subset of T-cells (T_{DTH}) reacting with antigen presented together with Class II MHC antigens produces lymphokines with diverse effects. These effects include macrophage chemotaxis, immobilization, and activation. At the onset of acquired immunity this may lead to systemic activation of macrophages. Local reactions lead to the local accumulation and activation of macrophages. There is evidence from many studies that tumor-associated antigens elicit immune responses of this sort. For example, typical cutaneous DTH reactions to tumor antigens have been elicited in appropriately immunized mice[66,67] and in some cancer patients.[68] Tests that detect T_{DTH} cells in vitro may also be positive. These include macrophage migration inhibition, leukocyte adherence inhibition,[69] and erythrocyte rosette augmentation.[70] Such tests have been found positive in tumor immune and tumor bearing mice[71] and patients with any of several common cancers, e.g., colon, breast, and melanoma.[72-75] The presence of circulating lymphokine-like activity[76] and the apparently spontaneous release of lymphokine[77] in some patients with malignant disease are also consistent with the operation of DTH.

In experimental animals, the ability to transfer tumor immunity is often vested in T-lymphocytes with the markers of T_{DTH} cells — Ly1$^+$2$^-$(3$^-$) in mice and W3/25$^+$ in rats.[78-81] Less directly, there is evidence for cell-mediated immunity* in the absence of cytotoxic T-cells.[82,83]

More evidence has been obtained in our laboratories for the involvement of DTH in

---

*   Although the evidence discussed in this section is consistent with and/or supports the idea that DTH is important in tumor immunity, other interpretations and possibilities are not excluded, e.g., that "T_{DTH}" cells may in fact be helper cells for other immune responses, as they possess similar markers to those on helper T-cells, or that cytotoxic T-cells (T_c) are important in the rejection of some tumors.

resistance to methylcholanthrene induced sarcomas in mice. In addition to the involvement of T$_{DTH}$ cells it was found that adoptive immunity required the participation of a noncommitted host cell with the characteristics of a macrophage.[84] As in DTH reactions, macrophages were found to accumulate locally in response to tumor antigens; this occurred in mice with concomitant immunity.[85] Resistance to tumor challenge could be depressed or totally abrogated by treatment of immune mice with agents that inhibited the expression of DTH: irradiation, niridazole, reserpine, or carrageenan.[86,87] Studies in rats again produced less clear-cut results. Irradiation depressed concomitant immunity to D8 and D8M, but not ST2, while carrageenan depressed concomitant immunity to D8 but not to D8M or ST2.[88]

The processes whereby macrophages become activated in the course of DTH reactions have been discussed in detail in several reviews.[71,78,80,90] It appears to be a multi-signal process, at least one signal being provided by macrophage activating lymphokine(s).[91] Interferon-γ seems to be the major macrophage activating factor, though it is not the only one.[92-96] Activated macrophages are able to recognize tumor cells as targets, but little appears to be known at the molecular level about the recognition process. In most studies contact has been required for destruction of the targets and several mechanisms of cytotoxicity have been proposed, notably the local production of a cytolytic protease.[38] In some experimental systems the local production of arginase, without cell contact, appeared to be an effective tumoricidal mechanism.[97,98]

Against the implication of DTH as a delivery and activation system must be set the ability of tumor cells to produce molecules which depress the expression of DTH and decrease macrophage mobility (see Section IV.). It may be that the postulated DTH reactions are sufficiently strong to overcome the effects of such tumor products. The accumulation of macrophages in tumors transplanted in thymus-deprived mice[99,100] suggests, however, that other mechanisms exist. One possibility is the production by tumors of substances chemotactic for macrophages.[101,102] The discordance between the reported production of chemotactic factors and factors depressing macrophage mobility has not been resolved.

Once within a growing tumor, macrophages may also kill tumor cells by means of ADCC, if an appropriate humoral antibody response has been made. Unlike antibody-independent cytotoxicity, ADCC by macrophages appears to depend on reactive oxygen intermediates. Mouse antibodies of the IgG2a isotype are particularly powerful mediators. The roles of antibodies and ADCC in immunity have been reviewed[31,103,104] but possibly deserve still more attention.

C. Significance

It might be expected that macrophages with cytotoxic potential would be important in reducing primary tumor growth and restricting metastases. Concomitant immunity in mice is associated with restriction of metastases (natural, artificial, or both.)[41,105-108] Arguments for the involvement of macrophages, T-cells and DTH have been presented above. They may, however, not be universally applicable. Gorelik et al.[109] reported that concomitant immunity was thymus-independent and, in contrast to the observations of Kearney and Nelson,[110] was always nonspecific. Niederkorn and Streilein[108] reported that concomitant immunity induced by a tumor in the anterior chamber of the eye was specific and thymus-dependent, but suggested that it did not involve DTH because they were unable to elicit DTH reactions to other antigens. In rats there was some relationship between concomitant immunity to a second tumor challenge in the foot and restriction of lung metastases, but it was not clear-cut.[88] In the case of dormant L5178Y cells in DBA/2 mice, macrophages seemed to be responsible for the maintenance of dormancy.[47]

The possibility that macrophages contribute to the restriction of tumor growth and spread must be considered against the background of two perennial problems in tumor immunology. First, many spontaneously arising tumors in experimental animals appear to be nonimmunogenic,[111-113] and it has proved difficult to demonstrate truly tumor-specific antigens in many human tumors.[114] Thus, many tumors might be considered unable to elicit either a powerful macrophage delivery and activation system in the form of DTH, or antibodies that might be involved in macrophage-mediated ADCC. Similarly, such tumors might also fail to trigger other defences, such as delivery systems for NK cells or the production of cytolytic T-cells. Second, many immunogenic tumors continue to grow despite the existence of demonstrable host immune responses.

The apparent lack of immunogenicity may be more apparent than real. For example, failure to detect immunity to spontaneous tumors in animals may be due to failure to test adequately for concomitant immunity. In cancer patients, apparently tumor-specific T-cells can be detected by means of an unconventional but well validated test, leukocyte adherence inhibition (see Section II.B.). Host immunity may be subverted, e.g., by tumor products which depress DTH and/or by the induction of suppressor cells[42,115] (Sections IV. and V.). The expression of cell-mediated immunity may be abrogated by soluble blocking factors of various sorts, including not only antibodies and antigen-antibody complexes,[116] but also immunologically specific nonimmunoglobulin factors,[117] host cell products such as immunoregulatory α-globulin[118] and other factors inhibiting nonspecific macrophage cytotoxicity.[119] Some macrophages may stimulate rather than inhibit tumor growth (Section III.). The net result for the host may depend largely on the balance between the rate of suppression of tumor cells (by activated macrophages or other cells) and the rate of proliferation of tumor cells (which may be increased by some macrophages). Thus, in concomitant immunity, the primary tumor isograft may reach a critical size at which its growth outstrips host suppressive mechanisms, while those same mechanisms can suppress small secondary challenges or metastases. As discussed by several workers, some host-tumor relationships may have elements of "a simple numbers game".[40,120,121]

III. TUMOR CELL STIMULATION BY MACROPHAGES

A. Occurrence

Perhaps the earliest suggestion that macrophages (or other host cells) might stimulate tumor growth came from an observation by Piessens et al.[122] They found that certain schedules of administration of BCG actually facilitated the growth of mammary carcinomas in rats, rather than depressing growth, as was expected of a macrophage stimulating, immunopotentiating agent. Similar observations were made on BCG cell walls in rats[123] and *Corynebacterium parvum* in mice.[124,125] Evans[126] found that a benzpyrene-induced fibrosarcoma grew less well in irradiated than in normal mice, the reduced growth being accompanied by a reduced macrophage content. Normal tumor growth could be restored, in irradiated mice, by mixing macrophages with the tumor inoculum.[127]

There are other examples of anti-inflammatory or "immunosuppressive" treatments leading to unexpected reductions in tumor growth in nonimmune animals. These include a treatment (before tumor inoculation) with irradiation,[128,129] corticosteroids,[129,130] cyclophosphamide,[129,131] and reserpine.[129,132] Reserpine has also been reported to inhibit the induction of cutaneous squamous cell carcinomas by methylcholanthrene in mice.[133] There are many ways in which these agents could interfere with host responses that are potentially beneficial to tumors, e.g., by inhibiting angiogenesis,[134] mast cell function,[135] or suppressor cell production.[131] One possibility is that macrophages potentiate tumor growth, as in the original experiments of Evans.

They might do this directly, by stimulating tumor cell proliferation, or indirectly in ways discussed in Sections IV and V.

There is considerable direct and indirect evidence that macrophages promote the proliferation of lymphoma cells in vitro.[136-139] Macrophages (or monocytes) have also been reported to increase the proliferation of virus-transformed mouse fibroblasts,[140] human myeloma cells,[141] various human epithelial tumor cells,[142] and a human cancer derived cell line.[143] It is noteworthy that tumor associated macrophages from human patients[144] and mice[145,146] stimulated proliferation of a variety of human and mouse tumor cells.

Our own experiments have been carried out with mouse sarcomas, both methylcholanthrene-induced and spontaneous.[147,148] Mixed cultures of normal resident peritoneal cells and tumor cells showed much greater incorporation of ³H-thymidine than did either cell type alone. The stimulation, which was not MHC-restricted, did not occur in mixtures of tumor cells and normal spleen cells, Chang cells, or fibroblasts. It did, however, occur in mixtures of tumor cells and peritoneal exudate cells induced by thioglycollate or proteose peptone. It also occurred in mixtures of tumor cells with peritoneal exudate cells induced by *C. parvum*, provided that the exudate cells were precultured for 48 hr to allow decay of their cytotoxicity.[149] Flow cytometry and autoradiography were used to help resolve the stimulation into two components. The minor component was stimulation of normal lymphocytes by a tumor cell product. The major component was stimulation of tumor cell proliferation by large adherent cells tentatively identified as macrophages. It as of great interest that clones of tumor cells, studied over a period of time, showed very marked cyclical variation in the degree of stimulation they underwent in mixed culture. This variation was unrelated to the density of the culture from which the tumor cells were obtained, the baseline ³H-thymidine incorporation by the tumor cells alone, or the frequency of passage of the cells in vitro.

Evidence for direct stimulation of tumor cell proliferation by macrophages in vitro is complemented by direct evidence of tumor growth promotion in vivo by macrophages. Evans[127] found that macrophages restored the growth of tumors in irradiated hosts. Kadhim and Rees[150] reported enhancement of the growth of subcutaneous transplants of syngeneic methylcholanthrene-induced tumors (but not lymphomas) by admixed macrophages; both resident peritoneal cells and tumor associated macrophages were effective. Gorelik et al.[151] found that thioglycollate-induced macrophages, injected intravenously, enhanced lung colony formation from B16 melanoma or Lewis lung carcinoma cells injected intravenously. Conversely, depletion of macrophages from inocula of rat tumors D8M and ST2 reduced their growth in the feet and, in the case of ST2, abolished local metastasis.[88]

B. Mechanisms

Little is known of the mechanisms of stimulation of tumor cell proliferation by macrophages. Where soluble products of macrophages stimulate lymphoma cells it might be surmised that IL-1, as a physiological signal, is at least partly responsible. Likewise, stimulation of malignantly transformed fibroblasts might be due to IL-1 or to other macrophage products which stimulate normal fibroblasts.[152,153] Trejdosiewicz et al.[143] found that monocyte supernatants were sometimes stimulatory. In our own experiments, however, no soluble mediator was detected and contact between macrophages and tumor cells appeared to be essential. The inhibition of stimulation by the protease inhibitor Trasylol and the direct stimulation of tumor cell proliferation by trypsin suggested that surface bound proteases of macrophages might be responsible in part. Stimulation in mixed cultures was, however, potentiated by 0.01 to 1 μM dexamethasone, which might be expected to inhibit proteases. It is conceivable that macrophages have the potential for two effects on tumor cells, stimulation and inhibition, and that dexamethasone interferes with their inhibitory capacity.[145] Gorelik et al.[151] found that disrupted macrophages enhanced lung colony formation; we have not done analogous experiments in vitro.

C. Significance

The ability of any host cell to potentiate tumor growth is clearly a source of unease. This is all the more so when cells present within a tumor can do so. Although this is not a universal phenomenon it may be more common than is suspected by many tumor biologists. The ability of macrophages to stimulate tumor cell proliferation may also be a powerful factor in the "immunostimulation of tumor growth", an idea eloquently expounded by Prehn.[154,155] It is possible that some potentiating tumor-associated macrophages are derived from macrophages that were initially cytotoxic but have lost this function. In this case, their sensitivity to signals stimulating cytotoxicity may have an important bearing on the outcome of attempted immunotherapy.

The cyclical changes in the susceptibility of cloned tumor cells to stimulation by macrophages[147] may be one reflection of the generation of variants, including the production of metastatic variants. It now seems likely not only that tumors consist of heterogeneous populations of cells and that metastases arise from variants,[156-158] but also that the heterogeneity — the formation of new variants — continues to develop within clones or metastases.[159-161] Cells that proliferate more extensively in the presence of host cells may have, during the evolution of a tumor, a selective advantage over other tumor cells. It is perhaps relevant also that tumor associated macrophages have been reported to be mutagenic[162] and that hybridization of a mouse lymphoma with normal macrophages led to the development of highly metastatic sub-lines.[163,164]

IV. OTHER FUNCTIONS OF THE MONONUCLEAR PHAGOCYTE SYSTEM

A. Monocytopoiesis

Monocytosis may accompany tumor carriage in man,[165] mice,[166,167] and rats.[168] After tumor transplantation in mice monocytopenia preceded monocytosis, and the macrophage colony forming capacity in vitro of bone marrow fell and rose in parallel.[166,167,169] A low molecular weight (less than 1000) tumor cell product, injected intravenously, depressed colony forming capacity; the depressive factor did not appear to be prostaglandin.[167] The mechanism of stimulation of monocytopoiesis is not known, but it is possible that colony stimulating factor(s) may be produced by stimulated lymphocytes and macrophages during a generalized cell-mediated immune response to tumor antigens (Section II.B.). The increased proliferation of resident peritoneal macrophages in tumor bearing mice is consistent with this view.[170]

B. Chemotaxis, Phagocytosis, and Inflammation*

In 1955 Rebuck and Crowley reported that the entry of monocytes into skin windows was depressed in cancer patients.[176] Dizon and Southam[177] made a similar observation. DTH reactions, in which immigrant monocytes are prominent, are also frequently depressed in patients with advanced cancer (reviewed by Burdick et al.[178]). Since the report by Hausman et al.[179] numerous studies have shown that monocytes from some cancer patients show depressed responses to chemotactic stimuli in vitro.[115,174,175] Tumor-bearing mice, rats, and guinea pigs also often have a depressed capacity to mount DTH reactions[180-183] and to mobilize macrophages in response to such nonspecific

---

* For more detailed discussions, see the reviews in References 115, 171 to 175.

stimuli as mineral oil,[180] glycogen,[181] proteose peptone,[184,185] phytohemagglutinin,[182,186] subcutaneous fibrous discs[185,187] and, in the original experiments of Fauve et al.,[188] fetal calf serum. In one study the depression was biphasic. There was a phase of depression shortly after transplantation of a lymphoma in mice or a fibrosarcoma in rats, followed by a period of normal activity, and later by the recurrence of depressed activity.[188a]

Most of the experimental studies have been carried out with transplanted tumors. Similar defects occurred in SJL/J mice developing spontaneous lymphomas[189] and in most AKR mice developing T-cell leukemia.[190] In mice and rats treated with methylcholanthrene, however, the relationship was unclear. There was some relationship between depression of macrophage accumulation and the subsequent development of tumors in both species. In rats the emergence of tumors was associated with some depression, but in neither species was the carriage of large autochthonous tumors associated with depression of macrophage accumulation. When transplanted to syngeneic recipients the same tumors did depress macrophage accumulation.[191] Ultraviolet light-induced tumors behaved similarly, but mammary tumor virus-induced tumors did not inhibit macrophage accumulation in either autochthonous hosts or syngeneic recipients.[192]

The overall phagocytic activity of macrophages of "the reticuloendothelial system" has been found to be increased in tumor-bearing mice.[1,166,171] Decreased activity was found early after tumor transplantation[166] and late in the course of tumor carriage.[171,172,174,193]

Many cancer patients have diminished resistance to infection, which may be related in part to their disease and, often, in part to treatment that has immunosuppressive effects. The contribution of defective macrophage function to the reduction in resistance is not known. In mice, systemic macrophage mediated resistance to *Listeria monocytogenes* was depressed shortly after syngeneic tumor transplantation;[194] resistance to proliferation within established tumors was also depressed.[195] Later in tumor growth, however, systemic resistance was increased,[196] a finding consistent with other evidence of macrophage stimulation, especially in mice with concomitant immunity. Tumor cells did not seem to impair the ability of mice to develop and express immunity to *Listeria* after immunization with an avirulent strain.[188]

C. Mechanisms of Tumor-Induced Changes

Mechanisms of changes in monocytopoiesis have been considered (Section IV.A.) The ways in which other changes in macrophage activity and inflammation are brought about may have a broader significance.

One of the pitfalls in studies of this sort is the contamination of mouse tumors by lactic dehydrogenase elevating virus (LDV). This widely distributed virus can cause many abnormalities in immune function,[197,198] including some abnormalities similar to those in tumor-bearing mice. Tumor-induced depression of macrophage mediated resistance to *Listeria* infection was attributed, in one study, to LDV.[199] Stevenson et al.[200] found that some tumors which caused an increase in macrophage phagocytic capacity and a decrease in chemotaxis contained LDV, and that injection of the virus alone or of serum from mice bearing infected tumors caused similar changes. However, such changes also occurred in mice bearing LDV-free tumors. LDV-free tumors and their products also caused inhibition of macrophage accumulation in vivo.[201] In our own experiments, tumors producing substances that depressed DTH reactions in mice had no lactic dehydrogenase elevating activity.[115] Although care should be exercised in evaluating their significance, many abnormalities are consequences of the carriage of malignant cells rather than of infection with passenger LDV.

Abnormalities of macrophage function could be produced in two general ways: as consequences of the interaction of the host immune system with tumor antigens; and by the direct action of tumor cell products. A widespread cell-mediated immune reaction could lead not only to macrophage activation (Section II.B.)., macrophage proliferation,[202] and increased monocytopoiesis (Section IV.A.), but also to increased macrophage phagocytic activity. On the other hand, tumor antigen-antibody complexes might be expected to reduce Fc receptor-mediated phagocytosis and antibody-dependent cell-mediated cytotoxicity by macrophages.[203] Immune complexes have been reported to inhibit the development and expression of macrophage tumoricidal capacity[204] and may have a more general immunosuppressive effect.[205,206]

Prostaglandins are produced by some tumors and may contribute to nonspecific immunosuppression[207] (Section V.A.) and, directly or indirectly, to the growth and spread of cancer.[208,209] PGE2 may contribute to the depression of monocytopoiesis (Section IV.A.). This seemed unlikely in our experiments, as indomethacin had no effect on the production of the inhibitor(s) of monocytopoiesis and some tumors producing the inhibitor(s) produced no detectable PGE2.[167] For similar reasons, prostaglandin was apparently not responsible for the depression by tumor products of phagocytosis by mouse macrophages.[210]

Macrophage mobility (spontaneous migration and chemotaxis) can be influenced by tumor cell products, as originally described by Fauve et al.[188] In some studies, inhibition of mobility was attributed to very low molecular weight (less than 1000) substances.[211,212] In others, soluble tumor products were found to have chemotactic or chemokinetic effects, usually on stimulated (peritoneal exudate) or activated macrophages.[101,102,213-215] Combination of stimulation of spontaneous migration and inhibition of chemotaxis has also been reported.[216] Monocyte polarization, a very early response to chemotactic stimuli in vitro, was inhibited by factors peculiar to human malignant effusions.[217] These factors had apparent molecular weights of 46,000 and 21,000 and reacted with monoclonal antibodies to the retrovirus envelope protein p15E (see below). A soluble tumor product(s) also depressed oxidative metabolism and the destruction of intracellular parasites (*Leishmania* and *Toxoplasma*) by activated mouse macrophages.[218] In our studies, tumor cell products inhibited hydrogen peroxide production by stimulated mouse and guinea pig macrophages, but not all tumor cells did so, while some normal cells did.[219]

Inhibition of macrophage mobility could provide a plausible explanation of the inhibition of macrophage accumulation in inflammatory responses (including DTH) in vivo. While this may well be a contributing factor, the inhibition of DTH at least seems to require further explanation, since (in our hands) tumor products of apparent molecular weight less than 1000 that inhibited migration in vitro did not inhibit DTH, and factors inhbiiting DTH (molecular weight greater than 1000) did not inhibit macrophage migration. Factors inhibiting DTH were glycoproteins, apparently of two broad classes: with apparent 1000 to 10,000 mol wt (L10) and greater than 10,000 (G10). L10 inhibited the early phase (24 hr) of DTH reactions of mice to sheep erythrocytes and G10 inhibited the late phase (30 hr onwards).[115,211] L10 was found to inhibit the production by stimulated lymphocytes of a lymphokine, macrophage chemotactic factor, and the production by macrophages of the monokine IL-1. Only mice more than 4-months-old appeared susceptible to the depression of DTH in vivo or the depression of lymphokine and monokine production in vitro. The production of IL-1 by activated macrophages was not inhibited.[220] The mode of action of G10 is unknown. In mice pretreated with low doses of cyclophosphamide, and thus putatively deprived of suppressor T-cells, DTH reactions were not inhibited.[293] This suggested the possibility that G10 (with or without L10) might depress DTH by an action on suppressor T-cells. Hersey et al.[221] reported that products of melanoma cells depressed IL-2 (but not IL-1) production by human peripheral blood mononuclear cells. We also have observed inhibition of IL-2 production by supernatants from cultures of mouse and human tumor cells, but not fibroblasts.[294] Much remains unclear in this area, e.g., the relationship of G10 to L10 — is it simply a polymer? — and the role of IL-2 in suppressor cell induction.[222-224] It is, however, conceivable that the depression of DTH involves inhibition of lymphokine production as a consequence of inhibition of IL-1 production and that the generation or operation of suppressor T-cells is favored by the absence of IL-2. Spleen cells from Balb/c mice bearing a fibrosarcoma produced less IL-2 than normal, and this was attributed to the presence of suppressor T-cells.[225] Inhibition of responsiveness to IL-2 has also been noted in the spleens of tumor-bearing mice[225] and in otherwise responsive normal cell populations exposed to tumor cell products.[226,294] Inhibition of IL-2 production or responsiveness (for whatever reason) could have further depressive effects on other cell mediated immune responses; this subject is further considered in Section V.A.

The relationship of soluble tumor products to the retrovirus envelope protein p15E is of special interest. As noted, inhibitors of monocyte polarization reacted with antibodies to p15E.[217] These antibodies also reduced or abolished the depression of DTH in mice by products of mouse and rat fibrosarcomas and of a bovine ocular squamous cell carcinoma (BOSCC).[227] p15E was detected in human cancer cells and mitogen transformed cells by means of flow cytometry.[228] At the least, antibodies to p15E should be useful in purifying the depressive factors, but the relationship of p15E to such factors may be of broader significance.

The possibility that soluble factors depressing host cell function are host cell products (e.g., prostaglandins, immunoregulatory α-globulin[118]) must also be kept in mind.

D. Significance

It is difficult to believe that defects in macrophage mobility, phagocytic capacity, and intracellular killing do not contribute to the susceptibility of cancer patients to infections. In several studies of monocyte chemotaxis a relationship was observed between the extent of disease and the degree of depression of chemotaxis. Not surprisingly there was also a relationship between the depression of chemotaxis and prognosis.[175]

The apparently universal production by tumor cells of factors depressing DTH suggests that this capacity might be a precondition for the emergence of overt malignancy. The relationship between these factors and inhibitors of monocyte polarization is not clear, but all those tested so far react with antibodies to p15E. It is possible that their production is governed by an oncogene-like entity, activation of which is an important factor in malignant transformation.[227,229] Consistent with this view are the appearance of antibodies to p15E in the sera of tumor immune mice,[230] the prevention of methylcholanthrene carcinogenesis in rats pretreated (? immunized) with a nontransforming retrovirus,[231] and a possible relationship between early mortality and the appearance of a retroviral protein (SiSV gp 70) in the circulation of patients with leukemia.[232]

It is also possible that factors depressing DTH and/or macrophage function could be targets of immunological intervention in cancer. BOSCC is sometimes susceptible to a form of immunotherapy: the injection of an adequate dose of a phenol-saline extract of an allogeneic BOSCC tumor often leads to partial or complete regression.[233] We have found that similar immunization of mice makes them resistant to the depression of DTH by saline extracts of BOSCC or by supernatants from rat mouse or human tumors. Antibodies to p15E also neutralize the depression of DTH. Immunization of mice with phenol saline extracts of allogeneic mouse tumor reduced the subsequent growth of syngeneic tumors in the feet.[227] These findings are consistent with the idea that resistance to the effects of tumor products resembling p15E may aid resistance to cancer.

A note of caution must, however, be sounded. In the experiments of Normann et al.[191,192] mice carrying primary tumors induced by chemicals, ultraviolet light or mammary tumor virus generally did not show defects in nonspecifically induced macrophage accumulation. It is, however, conceivable that these defects are unrelated to the depression of DTH, or that mice bearing primary tumors (which often grew more slowly than transplanted tumors) become resistant to the factors responsible. The relative susceptibility of old and young mice to the depression of DTH by tumor cell products also merits further investigation in relation to tumor susceptibility.

V. INTERACTIONS WITH OTHER CELLS AND TISSUES

A. T- and B-Cells: Suppressor Macrophages

Macrophages are commonly thought of as accessory cells in immune responses. The idea that they can act as suppressor cells has grown steadily since the 1960s when it was noted that excessive numbers of macrophages could inhibit primary antibody production in culture.[234,235] Later, macrophages were found to be at least partly responsible for the suppression of a variety of lymphoid cell responses in animals treated with macrophage activating agents, or with graft vs. host reactions, or bearing tumors (early work was summarized by Nelson[236] and Kirchner[237]). The subject of suppressor macrophages in cancer has recently been reviewed extensively and critically by Varesio[238] and only key points and critical issues will be summarized here.

Suppressive macrophages have been identified by quite stringent criteria in the lymphoid tissues (usually the spleen) of mice and rats bearing any of a wide variety of tumors. The development of suppressor macrophages does not seem to be related to the immunogenicity of a tumor. Less extensively, suppressor monocytes have been identified in patients with malignant disease. In general, T-cell responses or T-cell dependent responses are more markedly depressed than pure B-cell responses. A notable example, however, is myeloma, which is marked by defects in nonmalignant B-cell function. There appear to be two components to suppression by macrophages: suppression which can be brought about by normal macrophages or monocytes in increased numbers; and increased suppression (on a "per cell" basis) by stimulated or activated macrophages.

The relationship between activation (e.g., for tumoricidal activity) and development of suppressive activity is not clear. Populations of activated macrophages are usually also suppressive.[236,238] In one study, rat and mouse peritoneal cells activated by *C. parvum* were fractionated on the basis of size; the larger cells were both cytotoxic and suppressive.[239] On the other hand, Boraschi et al.[240] found that mice with genetic defects in the capacity to produce tumoricidal macrophages could still produce suppressor macrophages. Hengst et al.[241] noted a dissocation between suppressive activity and tumoricidal activity in pulmonary alveolar macrophages from patients with malignant or nonmalignant lung disease.

Suppressor macrophages can be induced in vitro by lymphokines;[242] this seems to be a step either distinct from or on the pathway to the induction of cytotoxic macrophages. Varesio[243] found that down regulation of RNA metabolism accompanied the development of cytotoxic, but not of suppressor, macrophages. On the other hand, Boraschi et al.[244] found that treatment with interferons (α, β, or γ) reduced the suppressive activity of normal macrophages, but they did not attempt to relate their observations to those of Varesio and his colleagues.

Other mechanisms can also operate to induce suppressor macrophages. A mouse myeloma product (molecular weight greater than 30,000) caused mouse peritoneal macrophages to produce a second factor depressing B-cell responses.[245] The work of Ting and his colleagues suggests that tumor cell products can directly induce suppressor macrophages which inhibit T-cell responses.[246-249] Macrophages suppressive of antibody production may also be induced by culture with tumor cells.[250]

In vitro, suppression by macrophages can be mediated by prostaglandins (mainly PGE2) and oxygen metabolites[251,252] or possibly by other factors.[245] A soluble tumor product has been reported to induce PGE synthesis in human monocytes.[253] PGE might have an immediate local suppressive effect, e.g., on T-cell proliferation and lymphokine production[254] and on the production of antibody to a thymus-dependent antigen.[250] It might also, however, have a long-term effect of wider significance by inhibiting IL-2 production and promoting suppressor T-cell formation.[255-257] For extensive discussions of the role of suppressor T-cells in tumor growth, the reader is referred to the reviews by Naor[258] and North.[42] In addition, PGE may have a down-regulating feedback effect on macrophage cytotoxicity.[259-260]

The significance of suppressor macrophages is to some extent open to question. In mice with suppressor macrophages, induced by chronic infection and detectable in vitro, DTH, allograft rejection and antibody production were normal.[261] This has been the case also in some, but not all, studies of tumor bearing mice.[238] The local action of suppressor macrophages either within a tumor or in the regional lymph nodes may well be more important than their systemic effect. Loss of the tumor dormant state in mice (see Section II.A.) was associated with the appearance of macrophages that suppressed cytolytic T-cell production, and this was of prognostic significance.[262] Studies of cancer patients have not revealed a clear relationship between the action of suppressor macrophages and disease extent or prognosis.[263,264] Perhaps, not surprisingly in view of the diversity of both tumor behavior and the effects of prostaglandins, indothemacin has had no consistent effect on tumor growth in mice.[207,265-267]

B. Other Cells and Systems

NK cells are discussed in detail elsewhere in this volume but it is appropriate to note here that macrophages can exert profound effects on NK cell activity. They may be involved in both the stimulation or maintenance of NK activity and in its inhibition, by way of PGE production.[268-271] Macrophages from mice with murine sarcoma virus induced tumors were suppressive of NK activity.[272]

Macrophage products also influence other mesenchymal cells which may be important in both primary tumor growth and metastasis. The development of an adequate blood supply is essential for tumor growth. While there is evidence that tumor cells can produce angiogenic factors[134] macrophages can also do so.[273-275] It is particularly relevant that macrophages isolated from rat tumors were able to induce both neovascularization in vivo and endothelial cell proliferation in vitro.[276] It should also be noted, however, that mast cells interact with tumor cells to stimulate endothelial cell proliferation in vitro.[277] The number of mast cells required to do this is very small and the possibility must be borne in mind that macrophage preparations might be contaminated by mast cells, which can and do infiltrate tumors.[278]

Other interactions between macrophages, tumor cells, endothelial, and other surfaces may be important. Rat macrophages have been reported to promote the attachment of tumor cells (in mixed cellular spheroids) to vascular endothelial cell monolayers in vitro.[279] Laminin can promote the attachment of metastatic tumor cells to basement membrane[280] but may also increase macrophage cytotoxicity.[281] Fibronectin, which may also promote the attachment of tumor cells, e.g., to connective tissue, has been reported to increase the cytotoxic and cytostatic effect of mouse macrophages.[282,283] By virtue of their production of IL-1[284] and other factors[285] that stimulate fibroblasts, macrophages may contribute to the development of a fibrous stroma. The ability of macrophages from tumor-bearing animals, particularly tumor-associated macrophages, to carry out these functions is worthy of further investigation.

A link between the clotting system and cancer has long been known. Evidence for the existence and importance of this link includes the presence of fibrin in tumors, the occurrence of clotting abnormalities in patients with cancer, and the inhibition of metastasis by treatment with anticoagulant drugs (reviewed by Rickles and Edwards[286]). Some tumor cells have direct procoagulant activity, but macrophages can also develop procoagulant activity in response to lymphokines and other stimuli,[287,288] including tumor cell products.[289] Thus, macrophages may contribute to the generation of fibrin in tumors and thereby perhaps to the establishment of metastases. Macrophages associated with rabbit tumors had strong procoagulant activity, as did circulating mononuclear cells from the same animals.[290] In mice, however, macrophages from weakly immunogenic tumors had normal or low levels of procoagulant activity and failed to respond to a further stimulant, LPS. On the other hand, macrophages from a highly immunogenic Moloney virus-induced tumor had high levels of procoagulant activity which did not rise further in response to LPS.[291] These intriguing but possibly discordant findings suggest that further studies would be rewarding. The ways in which fibrin might promote metastasis also deserve closer examination. Although it is commonly suggested that it assists by the formation of a surface or nest for tumor cells, it may also physically protect them from attack by NK cells.[292] Little is known, indeed, of the effects of fibrin on the interaction between target cells and macrophages delivered by means of a DTH reaction.

VI. CONCLUSION

One of the problems revealed by even a brief survey such as this is the difficulty of formulating "rules" which macrophages and tumor cells can be seen to obey. This stems from the diversity in behavior of both parties — the macrophages and the tumor cells. In particular, the very clear demonstrations that macrophages can sometimes stimulate tumor cell proliferation makes facile generalizations even more hazardous. Macrophages, in different guises, may promote or inhibit metastasis. The experimental tumor biologist is left in some awe of the subtlety and complexity of the balance between tumor cells, the immune system, macrophages and other cells and systems. It is to be hoped that this will not discourage vigorous attempts to utilize what is known in further studies of immunological intervention in cancer.

ACKNOWLEDGMENTS

The work of my laboratory referred to above has been supported by grants from the Australian National Health and Medical Research Council, the New South Wales State Cancer Council and the Postgraduate Medical Foundation of the University of Sydney, and by Research Contracts No 1-CB36973 and No 1-CB84251 from the National Cancer Institute. I thank Drs. John Wells and Peggy Nelson for helpful discussions and Mrs. Mary Cass for efficient preparation of the manuscript.

REFERENCES

1. Old, L. J., Benacerraf, B., Clarke, D. A., Carswell, E. A., and Stockert, E., The role of the reticuloendothelial system in the host reaction to neoplasia, *Cancer Res.*, 21, 1281, 1961.
2. Alexander, P. and Evans, R., Endotoxin and double stranded RNA render macrophages cytotoxic, *Nature (London) New Biol.*, 232, 76, 1981.

3. Hibbs, J. B., Jr., Lambert, L. H., Jr., and Remington, J. S., Possible role of macrophage mediated nonspecific cytotoxicity in tumour resistance, *Nature (London) New Biol.,* 235, 48, 1972.

4. Hibbs, J. B., Jr., Chapman, H. A., Jr., and Weinberg, J. B., The macrophage as an antineoplastic surveillance cell: biological perspectives, *J. Reticuloendothel. Soc.,* 24, 549, 1978.

5. Adams, D. O. and Snyderman, R., Do macrophages destroy nascent tumors?, *J. Natl. Cancer Inst.,* 62, 1341, 1979.

6. Keller, R., Regulatory capacities of mononuclear phagocytes with particular reference to natural immunity against tumors, in *Natural Cell-Mediated Immunity against Tumors,* Herberman, R. B., Ed., Academic Press, New York, 1980, 1219.

7. Fischer, D. G., Hubbard, W. A., and Koren, H. A., Tumor cell killing by freshly isolated peripheral blood monocytes, *Cell. Immunol.,* 58, 426, 1981.

8. Mantovani, A., Jerrells, T. R., Dean, J. H., and Herberman, R. B., Cytolytic and cytostatic activity on tumor cells of circulating human monocytes, *Int. J. Cancer,* 23, 18, 1979.

9. Mantovani, A., Polentarutti, N., Peri, G., Bar Shavit, Z., Vecchi, A., and Mangioni, C., Cytotoxicity on tumor cells of peripheral blood monocytes and tumor-associated macrophages in patients with ascites ovarian tumors, *J. Natl. Cancer Inst.,* 64, 1307, 1980.

10. Eggen, B. M. and Lamrik, J. O., Dissociation between cytostatic and cytolytic activity of human monocytes towards K562 cells, *Acta Pathol. Microbiol. Scand. Sect. C,* 92, 261, 1984.

11. Chang, Y. -H. and Yao, C. -S., Investigation of the human macrophage II. The in vitro cytotoxicity of macrophages, *Eur. J. Immunol.,* 9, 521, 1979.

12. Gerrard, T. L., Terz, J. J., and Kaplan, A. M., Cytotoxicity to tumor cells of monocytes from normal individuals and cancer patients, *Int. J. Cancer,* 26, 585, 1980.

13. Mantovani, A., Tagliabue, A., Dean, J. H., Jerrells, T. R., and Herberman, R. B., Cytolytic activity of circulating human monocytes on transformed and untransformed human fibroblasts, *Int. J. Cancer,* 23, 28, 1979.

14. Colotta, F., Peri, G., Villa, A., and Mantovani, A., Rapid killing of actinomycin D-treated tumor cells by human mononuclear cells. I. Effectors belong to the monocyte-macrophage lineage, *J. Immunol.,* 132, 936, 1984.

15. Kleinerman, E. S. and Herbeman, R. B., Tumoricidal activity of human monocytes: evidence for cytolytic function distinct from that of NK cells, *J. Immunol.,* 133, 4, 1984.

16. Horwitz, D. A., Knight, N., Temple, A., and Allison, A. C., Spontaneous and induced cytotoxic properties of human adherent mononuclear cells: killing of non-sensitized and antibody-coated non-erythroid cells, *Immunology,* 36, 221, 1979.

17. Cameron, D. J. and Churchill, W. H., Cytotoxicity of human macrophages for tumor cells: enhancement by lipopolysaccharide, *J. Immunol.,* 124, 708, 1980.

18. Normann, S. J. and Weiner, R., Cytotoxicity of human peripheral blood monocytes, *Cell. Immunol.,* 81, 413, 1983.

19. Nakahashi, H., Yasumoto, K., Nagashima, A., Yaita, H., Takeo, S., Motohiro, A., Furukawa, T., Inokuchi, K., and Nomoto, K., Antitumor activity of macrophages in lung cancer patients with special reference to location of macrophages, *Cancer Res.,* 44, 5906, 1984.

20. Kleinerman, E. S., Zwelling, L. A., Barlock, A., Young, R. C., Decker, J. M., Bull, J., and Muchmore, A. V., Defective monocyte killing in patients with malignancies and restoration of function during chemotherapy, *Lancet,* 2, 1102, 1980.

21. Cameron, D. J. and O'Brien, P., Cytotoxicity of cancer patients' macrophages for tumor cells, *Cancer,* 50, 498, 1982.

22. Cameron, D. J. and Stromberg, B. V., The ability of macrophages from head and neck cancer patients to kill tumor cells. Effect of prostaglandin inhibitors on cytotoxicity, *Cancer,* 54, 2403, 1984.

23. Kohl, S., Pickering, L. K., Sullivan, M. P., and Walters, D. L., Imparied monocyte-macrophage cytotoxicity in patients with Hodgkin's disease, *Clin. Immunol. Immunopathol.,* 15, 577, 1980.

24. De Young, N. J. and Gill, P. G., Monocyte antibody-dependent cellular cytotoxicity in cancer patients, *Cancer Immunol. Immunother.,* 18, 54, 1984.

25. Mantovani, A., Bar Shavit, Z., Peri, G., Polentarutti, N., Bordignon, C., Sessa, C., and Mangioni, C., Natural cytotoxicity on tumour cells of human macrophages obtained from diverse anatomical sites, *Clin. Exp. Immunol.,* 39, 776, 1980.

26. Lemarbre, P., Hoidal, J., Vesella, R., and Rinehart, J., Human pulmonary macrophage tumor cell cytotoxicity, *Blood,* 55, 612, 1980.

27. Bordignon, C., Avallone, R., Peri, G., Polentarutti, N., Mangioni, C., and Mantovani, A., Cytotoxicity on tumour cells of human mononuclear phagocytes: defective tumoricidal capacity of alveolar macrophages, *Clin. Exp. Immunol.,* 41, 336, 1980.

28. Kan-Mitchell, J., Hengst, J. C. D., Kempf, R. A., Rothbart, R. K., Simons, S. M., Brooker, A. S., Kortes, V. L., and Mitchell, M. S., Cytotoxicity of human pulmonary alveolar macrophages, *Cancer Res.,* 45, 453, 1985.

29. Nelson, D. S., Hopper, K. E., and Nelson, M., Role of the macrophage in resistance to cancer, in *The Handbook of Cancer Immunology,* Vol. 3, Waters, H., Ed., Garland STPM Press, New York, 1978, 107.

30. Pels, E. and Den Otter, W., Natural cytotoxic macrophages in the peritoneal cavity of mice, *Br. J. Cancer,* 40, 856, 1979.

31. Adams, D. O. and Hamilton, T. A., The cell biology of macrophage activation, *Ann. Rev. Immunol.,* 2, 283, 1984.

32. Ryning, F. W., Krahenbuhl, J. L., and Remington, J. S., Comparison of cytotoxic and microbicidal function of bronchoalveolar and peritoneal macrophages, *Immunology,* 42, 513, 1981.

33. Baker, H. J., Lindsey, J. R., and Weisbroth, S. H., Housing to contorl research variables, in *The Laboratory Rat,* Vol. 1, Baker, H. J., Lindsey, J. R., and Weisbroth, S. H., Eds., Academic Press, New York, 1979, 169.

34. Inoue, Y. and Nelson, D. S., Two anti tumour cytotoxic cells in the peritoneal cavity of rats: natural occurrence, augmentation and partial characterization, *Aust. J. Exp. Biol. Med. Sci.,* 60, 41, 1982.

35. Johnson, W. J. and Baylish, E., Tumor-cytotoxic activity of resident rat macrophages, *J. Reticuloendothel. Soc.,* 29, 369, 1981.

36. Hibbs, J. B., Jr., Taintor, R. R., Chapman, H. A., Jr., nd Weinberg, J. B., Macrophage tumor killing: influence of the local environment, *Science,* 197, 279, 1977.

37. Hopper, K. E., Harrison, J., and Nelson, D. S., Partial characterization of anti-tumor effector macrophages in the peritoneal cavities of concomitantly immune mice and mice injected with macrophage-stimulating agents, *J. Reticuloendothel. Soc.,* 26, 259, 1979.

38. Johnson, W. J., Somers, S. D., and Adams, D. O., Expression and development of macrophage activation for tumor cytotoxicity, in *Contemporary Topics in Immunobiology,* Vol. 13, Adams, D. O. and Hanna, M. G., Jr., Eds., Plenum Press, New York, 1984, 127.

39. Gray, J. D., Brooks, C. G., and Baldwin, R. W., Detection of either rapidly cytotoxic macrophages or NK cells in "activated" peritoneal exudates depends on the methods of analysis and the target cell type, *Immunology,* 42, 561, 1981.

40. Normann, S. J. and Cornelius, J., Cytokinetics of macrophage-mediated cytotoxicity, *Cancer Res.,* 44, 2313, 1984.

41. Gorelik, E., Concomitant immunity and the resistance to a second tumor challenge, *Adv. Cancer Res.,* 39, 71, 1983.

42. North, R. J., The murine antitumor immune response and its therapeutic manipulation, *Adv. Immunol.,* 35, 89, 1984.

43. Eccles, S. A. and Alexander, P., Immunologically mediated restraint of latent tumour metastases, *Nature (London),* 257, 52, 1975.

44. Gershon, R. K., Carter, R. L., and Lane, N. J., Studies on homotransplantable lymphomas in hamsters. IV. Observations on macrophages in the expression of immunity, *Am. J. Pathol.,* 51, 1111, 1967.

45. Wheelock, E. F., Weinhold, K. J., and Levich, J., The tumor dormant state, *Adv. Cancer Res.,* 34, 107, 1981.

46. Wheelock, E. F. and Robinson, M. K., Biology of disease. Endogenous control of the neoplastic process, *Lab. Invest.,* 48, 120, 1983.

47. Robinson, M. K. and Wheelock, E. F., Identification of macrophage-mediated cytolytic activity as a tumor-suppressive mechanism during maintenance of the L5178Y-tumor dormant state in DBA/2 mice, *J. Immunol.,* 126, 673, 1981.

48. Haskill, J. S., Proctor, J. W., and Yamamura, Y., Host responses within solid tumors. I. Monocytic effector cells within rat sarcomas, *J. Natl. Cancer Inst.,* 54, 387, 1975.

49. Haskill, J. S., ADCC effector cells in a murine adenocarcinoma. I. Evidence for blood-borne bone marrow-derived monocytes, *Int. J. Cancer,* 202, 432, 1977.

50. Vose, B. M., Cytotoxicity of adherent cells associated with some human tumours and lung tissues, *Cancer Immunol. Immunother.,* 5, 173, 1978.

51. Eccles, S. A. and Alexander, P., Macrophage content of tumours in relation to metastatic spread and host immune reaction, *Nature (London),* 250, 667, 1984.

52. Evans, R., Host cells in transplanted murine tumors and their possible relevance to tumor growth, *J. Reticuloendothel. Soc.,* 26, 427, 1979.

53. Nash, J. R. G., Puce, J. E., and Tarin, D., Macrophage content and colony-forming potential in mouse mammary carcinomas, *Br. J. Cancer,* 39, 478, 1981.

54. Key, M., Talmadge, J. E., and Fidler, I. J., Lack of correlation between the progressive growth of spontaneous metastases and their content of infiltrating macrophages, *J. Reticuloendothel. Soc.,* 32, 387, 1982.

55. Steele, R. J. C., Eremin, O., Brown, M., and Hawkins, R. A., A high macrophage content in human breast cancer is not associated with favourable prognostic factors, *Br. J. Surg.,* 71, 456, 1984.

56. Loveless, S. E. and Heppner, G. H., tumor-associated macrophages of mouse mammary tumors. I. Differential cytotoxicity of macrophages from metastatic and nonmetastatic tumors, *J. Immunol.*, 131, 2074, 1983.
57. Mahoney, K. H., Fulton, A. M., and Heppner, G. H., Tumor-associated macrophages of mouse mammary tumors. II. Differential distribution of macrophages from metastatic and nonmetastatic tumors, *J. Immunol.*, 131, 2079, 1983.
58. Wood, G. W. and Gillespie, G. Y., Studies on the role of macrophages in regulation of growth and metastasis of murine chemically induced fibrosarcomas, *Int. J. Cancer*, 16, 1022, 1975.
59. Inoue, Y. and Nelson, D. S., The effect of tumour-associated macrophages on the growth of tumours in rats, *Aust. J. Exp. Biol. Med. Sci.*, 62, 181, 1984.
60. Stewart, C. C., Local proliferation of mononuclear phagocytes in tumors, *J. Reticuloendothel. Soc.*, 34, 23, 1983.
61. Evans, R. and Cullen, R. T., In situ proliferation of intratumor macrophages, *J. Leuk. Biol.*, 35, 561, 1984.
62. Black, M. M., Kerpe, S., and Speer, F. D., Lymph node structure in patients with cancer of the breast, *Am. J. Pathol.*, 29, 505, 1953.
63. Nelson, D. S., *Macrophages and Immunity*, North-Holland, Amsterdam, 1968, 237.
64. Thoresen, S., Hartveit, F., Tangen, M., and Halvorsen, J. F., Sinus catarrh and histological grade in breast cancer, *Histopathology*, 7, 753, 1983.
65. Nelson, D. S., Macrophages as effectors of cell-mediated immunity, in *Phagocytes and Cellular Immunity*, Gadebusch, H. H., Ed., CRC Press, Boca Raton, Fla., 1979, 57.
66. Hoy, W. E. and Nelson, D. S., Delayed-type hypersensitivity in mice after skin and tumour allografts and tumour isografts, *Nature (London)*, 222, 1001, 1969.
67. Halliday, W. J. and Webb, M., Delayed hypersensitivity to chemically induced tumors in mice and correlation with an in vitro test, *J. Natl. Cancer Inst.*, 43, 141, 1969.
68. Herberman, R. B., Delayed hypersensitivity response toward autochthonous tumor extracts, *Recent Results Cancer Res.*, 47, 140, 1974.
69. Halliday, W. J. and Miller, S., Leukocyte adherence inhibition: a simple test for cell-mediated tumour immunity and serum blocking factors, *Int. J. Cancer*, 9, 477, 1972.
70. Maluish, A. E., Koppi, T. A., Harper, J. J., and Halliday, W. J., Augmentation of E-rosette formation by lymphocytes of cancer patients stimulated in vitro with tumour extracts, *Aust. J. Exp. Biol. Med. Sci.*, 58, 499, 1980.
71. Koppi, T. A. and Halliday, W. J., Further characterization of the cells involved in leukocyte adherence inhibition with murine tumor extracts, *Cell Immunol.*, 66, 394, 1982.
72. Halliday, W. J. Maluish, A., and Isbister, W. H., Detection of anti-tumour cell-mediated immunity and serum blocking factors in cancer patients by the leukocyte adherence inhibition test, *Br. J. Cancer*, 29, 31, 1974.
73. Grosser, N. and Thomson, D. M. P., Cell-mediated anti-tumor immunity in breast cancer patients evaluated by antigen-induced leukocyte adherence inhibition in test tubes, *Cancer Res.*, 35, 2571, 1975.
74. Winter, M., Nelson, D. S., and Milton, G. W., Leucocyte adherence inhibition test for the detection of cell-mediated immunity to malignant melanoma, *Aust. N.Z.J. Med.*, 10, 405, 1980.
75. Halliday, W. J., Koppi, T. A., Khan, J. M., and Davis, N. C., Leukocyte adherence inhibition: tumor specificity of cellular and serum-blocking reactions in human melanoma, breast cancer, and colorectal cancer, *J. Natl. Cancer Inst.*, 65, 327, 1980.
76. Cohen, S., Fisher, B., Yoshida, T., and Bettigole, R. E., Serum migration inhibitory activity in patients with lympho-proliferative diseases, *N. Engl. J. Med.*, 290, 882, 1974.
77. Waldman, R. H., Ganguly, R., and Cusumano, C. L., Spontaneous MIF secretion by peripheral lymphocytes of cancer patients, *J. Reticuloendothel. Soc.*, 23, 335, 1978.
78. Nelson, M., Nelson, D. S., McKenzie, I. F. C., and Blanden, R. B., Thy and Ly markers on lymphocytes initiating tumor rejection, *Cell. Immunol.*, 60, 34, 1981.
79. Fernandez-Cruz, E., Woda, B. A., and Feldman, J. D., Elimination of syngeneic sarcomas in rats by a subset of T lymphocytes, *J. Exp. Med.*, 152, 823, 1980.
80. Fernandez-Cruz, E., Gilman, S. C., and Feldman, J. D., Immunotherapy of chemically-induced sarcoma in rats: characterization of the effector T cell subset and nature of suppression, *J. Immunol.*, 128, 1112, 1982.
81. Robins, R. A. and Baldwin, R. W., T cell subsets in tumour rejection responses, *Immunol. Today*, 6, 55, 1985.
82. Lala, P. K. and McKenzie, I. F. C., An analysis of T lymphocyte subsets in tumor-transplanted mice on the basis of Lyt antigenic markers and functions, *Immunology*, 47, 663, 1982.
83. Stukart, M. J., Boes, J., and Melief, C. J. M., Immunity against Moloney sarcoma virus in H-2D^b mutant bm14 mice. Unimpaired tumor immunity despite absence of a virus-specific cytotoxic T cell response, *Int. J. Cancer*, 33, 265, 1984.

84. Simes, R. J., Kearney, R., and Nelson, D. S., Role of a non-committed accessory cell in the *in vivo* suppression of a syngeneic tumour by immune lymphocytes, *Immunology,* 29, 343, 1975.

85. Hopper, K. E. and Nelson, D. S., Specific triggering of macrophage accumulation at the site of secondary tumor challenge in mice with concomitant tumor immunity, *Cell. Immunol.,* 47, 163, 1979.

86. Nelson, M. and Nelson, D. S., Macrophages and resistance to tumors. II. Influence of agents affecting macrophages and delayed-type hypersensitivity on resistance to a tumor inducing specific "sinecomitant" immunity: acquired resistance as an expression of delayed-type hypersensitivity, *Cancer Immunol. Immunother.,* 4, 101, 1978.

87. Nelson, M. and Nelson, D. S., Macrophages and resistance to tumors. III. Influence of agents affecting macrophages and delayed-type hypersensitivity on resistance to tumors inducing concomitant immunity, *Aust. J. Exp. Biol. Med. Sci.,* 56, 211, 1978.

88. Inoue, Y. and Nelson, D. S., Modulation of natural and acquired immunity of rats to tumour isografts, *Aust. J. Exp. Biol. Med. Sci.,* 62, 167, 1984.

89. North, R. J., The concept of the activated macrophage, *J. Immunol.,* 121, 806, 1978.

90. Nathan, C. F., Murray, H. W., and Cohn, Z. A., The macrophage as an effector cell, *N. Engl. J. Med.,* 303, 622, 1980.

91. Meltzer, M. S., Tumor cytotoxicity by lymphokine-activated macrophages: development of macrophage tumoricidal activity requires a sequence of reactions, in *Lymphokines,* Vol. 3, Pick, E., Ed., Academic Press, New York, 1981, 319.

92. Ratliff, T. L., Thomasson, D. L., McCove, R. E., and Catalona, W. J., T-cell hybridoma production of macrophage activation factor (MAF). I. Separation of MAF from interferon gamma, *J. Reticuloendothel. Soc.,* 31, 393, 1982.

93. Schultz, R. M. and Kleinschmidt, W. J., Functional identity between murine γ interferon and macrophage activating factor, *Nature (London),* 305, 239, 1983.

94. Schreiber, R. D., Pace, J. L., Russell, S. W., Altman, A., and Katz, D. H., Macrophage activating factor produced by a T cell hybridoma. Physicochemical and biosynthetic resemblance to γ-interferon, *J. Immunol.,* 131, 826, 1983.

95. Krammer, P. H., Echtenbacher, B., Gemsa, D., Hamann, U., Hültner, L., Kaltmann, B., Kees, U., Kubelka, C., and Marcucci, F., Immune interferon (IFNγ), macrophage activating factors (MAFs), and colony-stimulating factors (CSFs) secreted by T cell clones in limiting dilution microcultures, long-term cultures, and by T cell hybridomas, *Immunol. Rev.,* 76, 5, 1983.

96. Nacy, C. A., James, S. L., Benjamin, W. R., Farrar, J. J., Hockmeyer, W. T., and Meltzer, M. S., Activation of macrophages for microbicidal and tumoricidal effector functions by soluble factors from EL-4, a continuous T cell line, *Infect. Immun.,* 40, 820, 1983.

97. Currie, G. A., Gyure, L., and Cifuentes, L., Microenvironmental arginine depletion by macrophages in vivo, *Br. J. Cancer,* 39, 613, 1979.

98. Farram, E. and Nelson, D. S., Mechanism of action of mouse macrophages as anti-tumor effector cells: role of arginase, *Cell. Immunol.,* 55, 283, 1980.

99. Szymaniec, S. and James, K., Studies on the Fc receptor-bearing cells in a transplanted methylcholanthrene-induced mouse fibrosarcoma, *Br. J. Cancer,* 33, 36, 1976.

100. Evans, R. and Eidlin, D. M., Macrophage accumulation in transplanted tumors is not dependent on host immune responsiveness or presence of tumor-associated rejection antigens, *J. Reticuloendothel. Soc.,* 30, 425, 1981.

101. Meltzer, M. S., Stevenson, M. M., and Leonard, E. J., Characterization of macrophage chemotaxis in tumor cell cultures and comparison with lymphocyte-derived chemotactic factors, *Cancer Res.,* 37, 721, 1977.

102. Bottazzi, B., Polentarutti, N., Balsari, A., Ghezzi, P., Salmona, M., and Mantovani, A., Chemotactic activity for mononuclear phagocytes of culture supernatants from murine and human tumor cells: evidence for a role in the regulation of the macrophage content of neoplastic tissues, *Int. J. Cancer,* 31, 55, 1983.

103. Shin, H. S., Johnson, R. J., Pasternack, G. P., and Economou, J. S., Mechanisms of tumor immunity: the role of antibody and nonimmune effectors, *Prog. Allergy,* 25, 163, 1978.

104. Adams, D. O., Cohen, M., and Koren, H. S., Activation of mononuclear phagocytes for cytolysis: parallels and contrast between activation for tumor cytotoxicity and for ADCC, in *Macrophage-Mediated Antibody-Dependent Cellular Cytotoxicity,* Koren, H. S., Ed., Plenum Press, New York, 1984, 155.

105. Kearney, R., Basten, A., and Nelson, D. S., Cellular basis for the immune response to methylcholanthrene-induced tumours in mice. Heterogeneity of effector cells, *Int. J. Cancer,* 15, 438, 1975.

106. Gorelik, E., Segal, S., and Feldman, M., Growth of a local tumor exerts a specific inhibitory effect on progression of lung metastases, *Int. J. Cancer,* 21, 617, 1978.

107. Janik, P., Bertram, J. S., and Szanlawska, B., Modulation of lung colony formation by a subcutaneously growing tumor, *J. Natl. Cancer Inst.,* 66, 1155, 1981.

108. Niederkorn, J. Y. and Streilein, J. W., Intracamerally induced concomitant immunity: mice harboring progressively growing intraocular tumors are immune to spontaneous metastases and secondary tumor challenge, *J. Immunol.*, 131, 2587, 1983.

109. Gorelik, E., Segal, S., and Feldman, M., On the mechanism of tumor "concomitant immunity", *Int. J. Cancer*, 27, 847, 1981.

110. Kearney, R. and Nelson, D. S., Concomitant immunity to syngeneic methylcholanthrene-induced tumors in mice. Occurrence and specificity of concomitant immunity, *Aust. J. Exp. Biol. Med. Sci.*, 51, 723, 1973.

111. Hewitt, H. B., Blake, E. R., and Walder, A. S., A critique of the evidence for active host defence against cancer, based on personal studies of 27 murine tumors of spontaneous origin, *Br. J. Cancer*, 33, 241, 1976.

112. Weiss, D. W., The questionable immunogenicity of certain neoplasms. What then the prospects for immunological intervention in malignant disease?, *Cancer Immunol. Immunother.*, 2, 11, 1977.

113. Middle, I. G. and Embleton, M. I., Naturally arising tumors of the inbred WBA/Not rat strain, II, Immunogenicity of transplanted tumors, *J. Natl. Cancer Inst.*, 67, 637, 1981.

114. Nelson, D. S., Human tumour immunology, *Aust. N.Z.J. Med.*, 9, 713, 1979.

115. Nelson, D. S., Nelson, M., Farram, E., and Inoue, Y., Cancer and subversion of host defences, *Aust. J. Exp. Biol. Med. Sci.*, 59, 229, 1981.

116. Hellström, K. -E., Hellström, I., and Nepom, J. T., Specific blocking factors — are they important?, *Biochim. Biophys. Acta Cancer*, 473, 121, 1977.

117. Koppi, T. A. and Halliday, W. J., Cellular origin of blocking factors from cultured spleen cells of tumor-bearing mice, *Cell. Immunol.*, 76, 29, 1983.

118. Cooperband, S. R., Badger, A. M., and Mannick, J. A., Non-hormonal serum suppressive factors, in *Mitogens in Immunobiology*, Oppenheim, J. J. and Rosenstreich, D. L., Eds., Academic Press, New York, 1976, 555.

119. Cameron, D. J. and Collawn, S. S., Cytotoxicity of cancer patients' macrophages for tumor cells: purification and characterization of plasma inhibitory factors obtained from colon cancer patients, *Int. J. Immunopharmacol.*, 5, 55, 1983.

120. Klein, G., Mechanisms of escape from immune surveillance, *Natl. Cancer Inst. Monograph*, 44, 135, 1976.

121. Nelson, D. S., Hopper, K. E., Blanden, R. V., Gardner, I. D., and Kearney, R., Failure of immunogenic tumors to elicit cytolytic T cells in syngeneic hosts, *Cancer Lett.*, 5, 61, 1978.

122. Piessens, W. F., Lachapelle, F. L., Legros, N., and Heuson, J. C., Facilitation of rat mammary tumour growth by BCG, *Nature (London)*, 228, 1210, 1970.

123. Wepsic, H. T., Alaimo, J., Druker, B. J., Murray, W., IV, and Morris, H. P., The negative systemic effect of BCGcw inoculated intraperitoneally. I. In vivo demonstration of intramuscular tumor growth enhancement with Morris hepatomas, *Cancer Immunol. Immunother.*, 10, 217, 1981.

124. Bomford, R., An analysis of the factors allowing promotion (rather than inhibition) of tumour growth by *Corynebacterium parvum*, *Int. J. Cancer*, 19, 673, 1977.

125. Peters, L. J., McBride, W. H., Mason, K. A., and Milas, L., A role for T lymphocytes in tumor inhibition and enhancement caused by systemic administration of *Corynebacterium parvum*, *J. Reticuloendothel. Soc.*, 24, 9, 1978.

126. Evans, R., Effect of X-irradiation on host-cell infiltration and growth of a murine fibrosarcoma, *Br. J. Cancer*, 35, 377, 1977.

127. Evans, R., Macrophage requirement for growth of a murine fibrosarcoma, *Br. J. Cancer*, 37, 1086, 1978.

128. Lerman, S. P., Carswell, E. A., Chapman, J., and Thorbecke, G. J., Properties of reticulum cell sarcomas in SJL/J mice. III. Promotion of tumor growth in irradiated mice by normal lymphoid cells, *Cell. Immunol.*, 23, 56, 1976.

129. Nelson, M., Nelson, D. S., and Hopper, K. E., Inflammation and tumor growth. I. Tumor growth in mice with depressed capacity to mount inflammatory responses: possible role of macrophages, *Am. J. Pathol.*, 104, 114, 1981.

130. Acero, R., Polentarutti, N., Bottazzi, B., Alberti, S., Ricci, M. R., Bizzi, A., and Mantovani, A., Effect of hydrocortisone on the macrophage content, growth and metastasis of transplanted murine tumors, *Int. J. Cancer*, 33, 95, 1984.

131. Glaser, M., Augmentation of specific immune response against a syngeneic SV40-induced sarcoma in mice by depletion of suppressor T cells with cyclophosphamide, *Cell. Immunol.*, 48, 339, 1979.

132. Scott, K. G., Scheline, R. R., and Stone, R. S., Mast cells and sarcoma growth in the rat, *Cancer Res.*, 18, 927, 1958.

133. Lupulescu, A., Reserpine and carcinogenesis: inhibition of carcinoma formation in mice, *J. Natl. Cancer Inst.*, 71, 1077, 1983.

134. Folkman, J., Angiogenesis: initiation and control, *Ann. N.Y. Acad. Sci.*, 401, 212, 1982.

135. Roche, W. R., Mast cells and tumors: the specific enhancement of tumor proliferation *in vitro, Am. J. Pathol.,* 119, 57, 1985.

136. Hersey, P. and Maclennan, I. C. M., Macrophage dependent protection of tumour cells, *Immunology,* 24, 385, 1973.

137. Nathan, C. F. and Terry, W. D., Differential stimulation of murine lymphoma growth *in vitro* by normal and BCG-activated macrophages, *J. Exp. Med.,* 142, 887, 1975.

138. Hewlett, G., Opitz, H. C., Flad, D. H. D., and Schlumberger, H. D., Macrophages/monocytes require cell-to-cell contact in order to regulate the growth of a murine lymphoma cell line, *J. Immunol.,* 123, 2265, 1979.

139. Umetsu, D. T., Lerman, S. P., and Thorbecke, G. J., Accessory cell requirements for lymphoma growth in vitro and in irradiated mice, *Cell. Immunol.,* 42, 139, 1979.

140. Goldman, R. and Bar-Shavit, Z., Dual effect of normal and stimulated macrophages and their conditioned media on target cell proliferation, *J. Natl. Cancer Inst.,* 63, 1009, 1979.

141. Salmon, S. E. and Hamburger, A. W., Immunoproliferation and cancer: a common macrophage-derived promoter substance, *Lancet,* 1, 1289, 1978.

142. Buick, R. N., Fry, S. E., and Salmon, S. E., Effect of host-cell interactions on clonogenic carcinoma cells in human malignant effusions, *Br. J. Cancer,* 41, 695, 1980.

143. Trejdosiewicz, L. K., Trejdosiewicz, A. J., Ling, N. R., and Dykes, P. W., Growth enhancing property of human monocytes from normal donors and cancer patients, *Immunology,* 37, 247, 1979.

144. Mantovani, A., Peri, G., Polentarutti, N., Bolis, G., Mangioni, C., and Spreafico, F., Effects on in vitro tumor growth of macrophages isolated from human ascitic ovarian tumors, *Int. J. Cancer,* 23, 157, 1979.

145. Mantovani, A., In vitro effects on tumor cells of macrophages isolated from an early-passage chemically-induced murine sarcoma and from its spontaneous metastases, *Int. J. Cancer,* 27, 221, 1981.

146. Evans, R., Duffy, T., and Cullen, R. T., Tumor-associated macrophages stimulate the proliferation of murine tumor cells surviving treatment with the oncolytic cyclophosphamide analogue ASTA 2-7557: in vivo implications, *Int. J. Cancer,* 34, 883, 1984.

147. Nelson, M. and Nelson, D. S., Stimulation of proliferation in mixed cultures of mouse tumor cells and nonimmune peritoneal cells. I. Occurrence of stimulation and cyclical variation in tumor cell activity, *J. Natl. Cancer Inst.,* 74, 627, 1985.

148. Nelson, M. and Nelson, D. S., Stimulation of proliferation in mixed cultures of mouse tumor cells and nonimmune peritoneal cells. II. Stimulation of tumor cells by macrophages and of lymphocytes by a tumor cell product, *J. Natl. Cancer Inst.,* 74, 637, 1985.

149. Nakamura, R. M. and Meltzer, M. A., Macrophage activation for tumor cytotoxicity: control of cytotoxic activity by the time interval effector and target cells are exposed to lymphokines, *Cell. Immunol.,* 65, 52, 1981.

150. Kadhim, S. A. and Rees, R. C., Enhancement of tumor growth in mice: evidence for the involvement of host macrophages, *Cell Immunol.,* 87, 259, 1984.

151. Gorelik, E., Wiltrout, R. H., Brunda, M. J., Holden, H. T., and Herberman, R. B., Augmentation of metastasis formation by thioglycollate elicited macrophages, *Int. J. Cancer,* 29, 575, 1982.

152. Schmidt, J. A., Mizel, S. B., Cohen, D., and Green, I., Interleukin 1, a potential regulator of fibroblast proliferation, *J. Immunol.,* 128, 2177, 1982.

153. Dohlman, J. G., Payan, D. G., and Goetzl, E. J., Generation of a unique fibroblast-activating factor by human monocytes, *Immunology,* 52, 577, 1984.

154. Prehn, R. T., Immunostimulation of the lymphodependent phase of neoplastic growth, *J. Natl. Cancer Int.,* 59, 1043, 1977.

155. Prehn, R. T., The dose-response curve in tumor-immunity, *Int. J. Immunopharmacol.,* 5, 255, 1983.

156. Poste, G. and Fidler, I. J., The pathogenesis of cancer metastasis, *Nature (London),* 283, 139, 1980.

157. Albino, A. P., Le Strange, R., Oliff, A. I., Furth, M. E., and Old, L. J., Transforming ras genes from human melanoma: a manifestation of tumour heterogeneity?, *Nature (London),* 308, 69, 1984.

158. Heppner, G. H., Tumor heterogeneity, *Cancer Res.,* 44, 2259, 1984.

159. Poste, G., Tzeng, J., Doll, J., Greig, R., Rieman, D., and Zeidman, I., Evolution of tumor cell heterogeneity during progressive growth of individual lung metastases, *Proc. Natl. Acad. Sci. U.S.A.,* 79, 6574, 1982.

160. Sweeney, F. L., Pot-Deprun, J., Poupon, M.-F., and Chouroulnikov, I., Heterogeneity of the growth and metastatic behaviour of cloned cell lines derived from a primary rhabdomyosarcoma, *Cancer Res.,* 42, 3776, 1982.

161. Chow, D. A., Ray, M., and Greenberg, A. H., In vivo generation and selection of variants with altered sensitivity to natural resistance (NR): a model of tumor progression, *Int. J. Cancer,* 31, 99, 1983.

162. Fulton, A. M., Loveless, S. E., and Heppner, G. H., Mutagenic activity of tumor-associated macrophages in *Salmonella typhimurium* strains TA98 and TA100, *Cancer Res.,* 44, 4308, 1984.

163. Larizza, L., Schirrmacher, V., and Pflüger, E., Acquisition of high metastatic capacity after in vitro fusion of a nonmetastatic tumor line with a bone marrow-derived macrophage, *J. Exp. Med.,* 160, 1579, 1984.

164. Larizza, L., Schirrmacher, V., Graf, L., Pflüger, E., Peres-Martinez, M., and Stöhr, M., Suggestive evidence that the highly metastic variant ESb of the T-cell lymphoma Eb is derived from spontaneous fusion with a host macrophage, *Int. J. Cancer,* 34, 699, 1984.

165. Territo, M. and Cline, M. J., Macrophages and their disorders in man, in *Immunobiology of the Macrophage,* Nelson, D. S., Ed., Academic Press, New York, 1976, 593.

166. Otu, A. A., Russell, R. J., Wilkinson, P. C., and White, R. G., Alterations of mononuclear phagocyte function induced by Lewis lung carcinoma in C57Bl mice, *Br. J. Cancer,* 36, 330, 1977.

167. Farram, E., Nelson, M., and Nelson, D. S., Macrophages and resistance to tumors. The effects of tumor cell products on monocytopoiesis, *J. Reticuloendothel. Soc.,* 30, 259, 1981.

168. Eccles, S. A., Bandlow, G., and Alexander, P., Monocytosis associated with the growth of transplanted syngeneic rat sarcomata differing in immunogenicity, *Br. J. Cancer,* 34, 20, 1976.

169. Baum, M. and Fisher, B., Macrophage production by the bone marrow of tumor-bearing mice, *Cancer Res.,* 32, 2813, 1972.

170. Nelson, D. S. and Kearney, R., Macrophages and lymphoid tissues in mice with concomitant tumor immunity, *Br. J. Cancer,* 34, 221, 1976.

171. Levy, M. H. and Wheelock, E. F., The role of macrophages in defense against neoplastic disease, *Adv. Cancer Res.,* 20, 131, 1974.

172. Kamo, I. and Friedman, H., Immunosuppression and the role of suppressive factors in cancer, *Adv. Cancer Res.,* 25, 271, 1977.

173. North, R. J., Spitalny, G. L., and Kirstein, D. P., Antitumor defense mechanisms and their subversion, in *The Handbook of Cancer Immunology,* Vol. 2, Waters, H., Ed., Garland STPM Press, New York, 1978, 187.

174. Stern, K., Control of tumors by the RES, in *The Reticuloendothelial System, Vol. 5, Cancer,* Herberman, R. B. and Friedman, H., Eds., Plenum Press, New York, 1983, 59.

175. Cianciolo, G. J. and Snyderman, R., Neoplasia and mononuclear phagocyte function, in The Reticulendothelial System, Vol. 5, Herberman, R. B. and Friedman, H., Eds., Plenum Press, New York, 1983, 193.

176. Rebuck, J. W. and Crowley, J. H., A method of studying leukocytic functions in vivo, *Ann. N.Y. Acad. Sci.,* 59, 757, 1955.

177. Dizon, Q. S. and Southam, C. M., Abnormal cellular reponse to skin abrasion in cancer patients, *Cancer,* 16, 1288, 1963.

178. Burdick, J. F., Wells, S. A., Jr., and Herberman, R. B., Immunologic evaluation of patients with cancer by delayed hypersensitivity reactions, *Surg. Gynecol. Obstet.,* 141, 779, 1975.

179. Hausman, M., Brosman, S., Fahey, J. L., and Snyderman, R., Defective mononuclear leukocyte chemotactic activity in patients with genitourinary carcinoma, *Clin. Res.,* 21, 646A, 1973.

180. Bernstein, I. D., Zbar, B., and Rapp, H. J., Impaired inflammatory response in tumor-bearing guinea pigs, *J. Natl. Cancer Inst.,* 49, 1641, 1972.

181. Eccles, S. A. and Alexander, F., Sequestration of macrophages in growing tumours and its effects on the immunological capacity of the host, *Br. J. Cancer,* 30, 42, 1974.

182. Wells, J. H., Cain, W. A., Wells, R. S., and Bozalis, J. R., Suppression of tuberculin and phytohaemagglutinin skin tests by large tumours in inbred mice, *Int. Arch. Allergy,* 47, 362, 1974.

183. Jessup, J. M., Cohen, M. H., Tomaszewski, M. M., and Felix, E. L., Effects of murine tumors on delayed hypersensitivity to dinitrochlorobenzene. I. Description of anergy caused by transplanted tumors, *J. Natl. Cancer Inst.,* 57, 1077, 1976.

184. Normann, S. J. and Sorkin, E., Cell-specific defect in monocyte function during tumor growth, *J. Natl. Cancer Inst.,* 57, 135, 1976.

185. Normann, S. J. and Cornelius, J., Concurrent depression of tumor macrophage infiltration and systemic inflammation by progressive cancer growth, *Cancer Res.,* 38, 3453, 1978.

186. Snyderman, R., Pike, M. C., Blaylock, B. L., and Weinstein, P., Effects of neoplasms on inflammation: depression of macrophage accumulation after tumor implantation, *J. Immunol.,* 116, 585, 1976.

187. Normann, S. J., and Schardt, M., A cancer related macrophage dysfunction in inflamed tissues, *J. Reticuloendothel. Soc.,* 24, 147, 1978.

188. Fauve, R. M., Hevin, B., Jacob, H., Gaillard, J. A., and Jacob, F., Anti-inflammatory effects of murine malignant cells, *Proc. Natl. Acad. Sci. U.S.A.,* 71, 4052, 1974.

188a. Normann, S. J., Schardt, M., and Sorkin, E., Biphasic depression of macrophage function after tumor transplantation, *Int. J. Cancer,* 28, 185, 1981.

189. Normann, S. J., Schardt, M., and Sorkin, E., Anti-inflammatory effect of spontaneous lymphoma in SJL/J mice, *J. Natl. Cancer Inst.,* 63, 825, 1979.

190. Normann, S. J., Schardt, M., and Sorkin, E., Alteration of macrophage function in AKR leukemia, *J. Natl. Cancer Inst.*, 66, 157, 1981.
191. Normann, S. J., Schardt, M. C., and Sorkin, E., Macrophage inflammatory responses in rats and mice with autochthonous and transplanted tumors induced by 3-methylcholanthrene, *J. Natl. Cancer Inst.*, 72, 175, 1984.
192. Normann, S. J., Schardt, M. C., and Sorkin, E., Authochthonous murine tumors: effects of viral or ultraviolet induction, immunogenicity and transplantation on intratumoral macrophages and systemic inflammatory responses, *Eur. J. Clin. Oncol.*, 21, 119, 1985.
193. Blamey, R. W., Crosby, D. L., and Baker, J. M., Reticuloendothelial activity during the growth of rat sarcomas, *Cancer Res.*, 29, 335, 1969.
194. North, R. J., Kirstein, D. P., and Tuttle, R. L., Subversion of host defense mechanisms by murine tumors. I. A circulating factor that suppresses macrophage-mediated resistance to infection, *J. Exp. Med.*, 143, 559, 1976.
195. Spitalny, G. L. and North, R. J., Subversion of host defence mechanisms by malignant tumors: an established tumor as a privileged site for bacterial growth, *J. Exp. Med.*, 154, 1264, 1977.
196. North, R. J., Kirstein, D. P., and Tuttle, R. L., Subversion of host defense mechanisms by murine tumors. II. Counter-influence of concomitant tumor immunity, *J. Exp. Med.*, 143, 574, 1976.
197. Notkins, A. L., Enzymatic and immunologic alterations in mice infected with lactic dehydrogenase virus, *Am. J. Pathol.*, 64, 733, 1971.
198. Riley, V., Spackman, D. H., Santisteban, G. A., Dalldorf, G., Hellström, I., Hellström, K. E., Lance, E. M., Rowson, K. E. K., Mahy, B. W. J., Alexander, P., Stock, C. C., Sjögren, H. O., Hollander, V. P., and Horzinek, M. C., The LDH virus: an interfering biological contaminant, *Science*, 200, 124, 1978.
199. Bonventre, P. F., Bubel, H. C., Michael, J. G., and Nickol, A. D., Impaired resistance to bacterial infection after tumor implant is traced to lactic dehydrogenase virus, *Infect. Immun.*, 30, 316, 1980.
200. Stevenson, M. M., Rees, J. C., and Meltzer, M. S., Macrophage function in tumor-bearing mice: evidence for lactic dehydrogenase-elevating virus-associated changes, *J. Immunol.*, 124, 2892, 1980.
201. Snyderman, R. and Cianciolo, G. J., Further studies of a macrophage chemotaxis inhibitor (MCI) produced by murine neoplasms: murine tumors free of lactic dehydrogenase virus produce MCI, *J. Reticuloendothel. Soc.*, 26, 453, 1979.
202. More, D. G., Penrose, J. M., Kearney, R., and Nelson, D. S., Immunological induction of DNA synthesis in mouse peritoneal macrophages. An expression of cell-mediated immunity, *Int. Arch. Allergy*, 44, 611, 1973.
203. Robins, R. A. and Baldwin, R. W., Immune complexes in cancer, *Cancer Immunol. Immunother.*, 4, 1, 1978.
204. Esparza, I., Green, R., and Schreiber, R. D., Inhibition of macrophage tumoricidal activity by immune complexes and altered erythrocytes, *J. Immunol.*, 131, 2117, 1983.
205. Specter, S. and Friedman, H., Immunosuppressive factors produced by tumors and their effects on the RES, in *The Reticuloendothelial System*, Vol. 5, Herberman, R. B. and Friedman, H., Eds., Plenum Press, New York, 1983, 315.
206. Abbas, A. K. and Klaus, G. G. B., Antibody-antigen complexes suppress antibody production by mouse plasmacytoma cells in vitro, *Eur. J. Immunol.*, 8, 217, 1978.
207. Plescia, O. J., Smith, A., and Grinwich, K., Subversion of immune system by tumor cells and role of prostaglandins, *Proc. Natl. Acad. Sci. U.S.A.*, 72, 1848, 1975.
208. Easty, G. C. and Easty, D. M., Prostaglandins and cancer, *Cancer Treat. Rev.*, 3, 217, 1976.
209. Goodwin, J. S., Husby, G., and Williams, R. C., Jr., Prostaglandin E and cancer growth, *Cancer Immunol. Immunother.*, 8, 3, 1980.
210. Nelson, M. and Nelson, D. S., Macrophages and resistance to tumors. VI. The effects of supernatants from cultures of normal and tumor cells on phagocytosis, *J. Reticuloendothel. Soc.*, 31, 433, 1982.
211. Nelson, M. and Nelson, D. S., Macrophages and resistance to tumors. IV. Influence of age on susceptibility of mice to anti-inflammatory and antimacrophage effects of tumor cell products, *J. Natl. Cancer Inst.*, 65, 781, 1980.
212. Warabi, H., Venkat, K., Geetha, V., Liotta, L. A., Brownstein, M., and Schiffmann, E., Identification and partial characterization of a low-molecular-weight inhibitor of leukotaxis from fibrosarcoma cells, *Cancer Res.*, 44, 915, 1984.
213. Snodgrass, M. J., Harris, T. M., and Kaplan, A. M., Chemokinetic response of activated macrophages to soluble products of neoplastic cells, *Cancer Res.*, 38, 2925, 1978.
214. Schaub Simon, L., Patterson, R., and Jones, T. L., A rapid method for assessment of a macrophage chemoattractant produced by SaD2 fibrosarcoma cells in vitro, *J. Immunol. Methods*, 32, 195, 1980.
215. Lane, R. D., Kaplan, A. M., Snodgrass, M. J., Spriggs, D. J., and Szakal, A. K., Localization of a macrophage chemokinetic factor on neoplastic cells, *J. Natl. Cancer Inst.*, 72, 871, 1984.

216. Young, M. R., Sundharadas, G., Cantarow, W. D., and Kumar, P. R., Purification and functional characterization of a low molecular weight immune modulating factor produced by Lewis lung carcinoma, *Int. J. Cancer*, 30, 517, 1982.

217. Cianciolo, G., Hunter, J., Silva, J., Haskill, J. S., and Snyderman, R., Inhibitors of monocyte responses to chemotaxins are present in human cancerous effusions and react with monoclonal antibodies to the p15(E) structural protein of retroviruses, *J. Clin. Invest.*, 68, 831, 1981.

218. Szuro-Sudol, A., Murray, H. W., and Nathan, C. F., Suppression of macrophage antimicrobial activity by a tumor cell product, *J. Immunol.*, 131, 384, 1983.

219. Nelson, M., Booth, M. L., and Nelson, D. S., Effect of tumour cell culture superantants on some biochemical activities of macrophages, *Aust. J. Exp. Biol. Med. Sci.*, 60, 493, 1982.

220. Farram, E., Nelson, M., Nelson, D. S., and Moon, D. K., Inhibition of cytokine production by a tumour cell product, *Immunology*, 46, 603, 1982.

221. Hersey, P., Bindon, C., Czerniecki, M., Spurling, A., Wass, J., and McCarthy, W. H., Inhibition of interleukin 2 production by factors released from tumor cells, *J. Immunol.*, 131, 2837, 1983.

222. Ting, C.-C., Yang, S. S., and Hargrove, M. E., Induction of suppressor T cells by interleukin 2, *J. Immunol.*, 133, 261, 1984.

223. Thoman, M. L. and Weigle, W. O., Interleukin 2 induction of antigen-nonspecific suppressor cells, *Cell. Immunol.*, 85, 215, 1984.

224. Malkovský, M. and Medawar, P. B., Is immunological tolerance (non-responsiveness) a consequence of interleukin 2 deficit during the recognition of antigen?, *Immunol. Today*, 5, 340, 1984.

225. Burger, C. J., Elgert, K. D., and Farrar, W. L., Interleukin 2 (IL-2) activity during tumor growth: IL-2 production kinetics, absorption of and responses to exogenous IL-2, *Cell. Immunol.*, 84, 228, 1984.

226. Fontana, A., Hengartner, H., De Tribolet, N., and Weber, E., Glioblastoma cells release interleukin 1 and factors inhibiting interleukin 2-mediated effects, *J. Immunol.*, 132, 1837, 1984.

227. Nelson, M., Nelson, D. S., Spradbrow, P. B., Kuchroo, V. K., Jennings, P. A., Cianciolo, G. J., and Snyderman, R., Successful tumour immunotherapy: possible role of antibodies to anti-inflammatory factors produced by neoplasms, *Clin. Exp. Immunol.*, 61, 109, 1985.

228. Cianciolo, G. J., Phipps, D., and Snyderman, R., Human malignant and mitogen-transformed cells contain retroviral p15E-related antigen, *J. Exp. Med.*, 159, 964, 1984.

229. Snyderman, R. and Cianciolo, G. J., Immunosuppressive activity of the retroviral envelope protein p15E and its possible relationship to neoplasia, *Immunol. Today*, 5, 240, 1984.

230. Klitzman, J. M., Brown, J. P., Hellström, K. E., and Hellström, I., Antibodies to murine leukemia virus gp70 and p15(E) in sera of Balb/c mice immunized with syngeneic chemically induced sarcomas, *J. Immunol.*, 124, 2552, 1980.

231. Fish, D. C., Demarais, J. T., Djurickovic, D., and Huebner, R. J., Prevention of 3-methylcholanthrene-induced fibrosarcomas in rats pre-inoculated with endogenous rat retrovirus, *Proc. Natl. Acad. Sci. U.S.A.*, 78, 2526, 1981.

232. Hehlmann, R., Erfle, V., Schetters, H., Luz, A., Rohmer, H., Schreiber, M. A., Pralle, H., Essers, U., and Weber, W., Antigens and circulating immune complexes related to the primate retroviral glycoprotein SiSV gp70. Indicators of early mortality in human acute leukemias and chronic myelogenous leukemias in blast crisis, *Cancer*, 54, 2927, 1984.

233. Spradbrow, P. B., Wilson, B. E., Hoffman, D., Kelly, W. R., and Francis, J., Immunotherapy of bovine ocular squamous cell carcinomas, *Vet. Rec.*, 100, 376, 1977.

234. Perkins, E. and Makinodan, T., The suppressive role of mouse peritoneal phagocytes in agglutinin response, *J. Immunol.*, 94, 767, 1965.

235. Mishell, R. I. and Dutton, R. W., Immunization of dissociated spleen cell cultures from normal mice, *J. Exp. Med.*, 126, 423, 1967.

236. Nelson, D. S., Nonspecific immunoregulation by macrophages and their products, in *Immunology of the Macrophage*, Nelson, D. S., Ed., Academic Press, New York, 1976, 235.

237. Kirchner, H., Suppressor cells of immune reactivity in malignancy, *Eur. J. Cancer*, 14, 453, 1978.

238. Varesio, L., Suppressor cells and cancer: inhibition of immune functions by macrophages, in *The Reticuloendothelial System*, Vol. 5, Herberman, R. B. and Friedman, H., Eds., Plenum Press, New York, 1983, 217.

239. Miller, G. A. and Morahan, P. S., Functional and biochemical heterogeneity among subpopulations of rat and mouse peritoneal macrophages, *J. Reticuloendothel. Soc.*, 32, 111, 1982.

240. Boraschi, D., Pasqualetto, D., Ghezzi, P., Salmona, M., Bartalina, M., Barbarulli, G., Censini, S., Soldateschi, D., and Tagliabue, A., Dissociation between macrophage tumoricidal capacity and suppressive activity: analysis with macrophage-defective mouse strains, *J. Immunol.*, 131, 1707, 1983.

241. Hengst, J. C. D., Kan-Mitchell, J., Kempf, R. A., Strumpf, I. J., Sharma, O. P., Kortes, V. L., and Mitchell, M. S., Correlation between cytotoxic and suppressor activities of human pulmonary alveolar macrophages, *Cancer Res.*, 45, 459, 1985.

242. Taramelli, D., Holden, H. T., and Varesio, L., In vitro induction of tumoricidal and suppressor macrophages by lymphokines: possible feedback regulation, *J. Immunol.*, 126, 2123, 1981.
243. Varesio, L., Down regulation of RNA labeling as a selective marker for cytotoxic but not suppressor macrophages, *J. Immunol.*, 132, 2683, 1984.
244. Borachi, D., Censini, S., and Tagliabue, A., Interferon-γ reduces macrophage-suppressive activity by inhibiting prostaglandin E2 release and inducing interleukin 1 production, *J. Immunol.*, 133, 764, 1984.
245. Kennard, J. and Zolla-Pasner, S., Origin and function of suppressor macrophages in myeloma, *J. Immunol.*, 124, 268, 1980.
246. Ting, C.-C. and Rodrigues, D., Reversal by peritoneal adherent cells of tumor cell suppression of T cell-mediated immunity, *J. Immunol.*, 123, 801, 1979.
247. Ting, C.-C. and Rodrigues, D., Immunoregulatory circuit among macrophage subsets for T cell-mediated cytotoxic response to tumor cells, *J. Immunol.*, 124, 1039, 1980.
248. Ting, C-C. and Rodrigues, D., Increased susceptibility to tumor cell immunosuppressive effect in tumor-bearing mice, *J. Natl. Cancer Inst.*, 65, 205, 1980.
249. Ting, C-C., Rodrigues, D., Ting, R. C., Wivel, N., and Collins, M. J., Suppression of T cell-mediated immunity by tumor cells: immunogenicity versus immunosuppression and preliminary characterization of suppressive factors, *Int. J. Cancer*, 24, 644, 1979.
250. Plescia, O. J., Pontieri, G. M., Brown, J., Racis, S., Ippoliti, F., Bellelli, L., Sezzi, M. L., and Lipari, M., Amplification by macrophages of prostaglandin-mediated immunosuppression in mice bearing syngeneic tumors, *Prostaglandins, Leuk. Med.*, 16, 205, 1984.
251. Metzger, Z., Hoffeld, J. T., and Oppenheim, J. J., Macrophage-mediated suppression. I. Evidence for participation of both hydrogen peroxide and prostaglandins in suppression of murine lymphocyte proliferation, *J. Immunol.*, 124, 983, 1980.
252. Hoffeld, J. T., Metzger, Z., and Oppenheim, J. J., Oxygen-derived metabolites as suppressors of immune responses in vitro, in *Lymphokines*, Vol. 2, Pick, E., Ed., Academic Press, New York, 1981, 63.
253. Leung, K. H., Fischer, D. G., and Koren, H. S., Erythromyeloid tumor cells (K562) induce PGE synthesis in human peripheral blood monocytes, *J. Immunol.*, 131, 445, 1983.
254. Stenson, W. F. and Parker, C. W., Prostaglandins, marcrophages and immunity, *J. Immunol.*, 125, 1, 1980.
255. Nicklin, S. and Shand, F. L., Abrogation of suppressor cell function by inhibitors of prostaglandin synthesis, *Int. J. Immunopharmacol.*, 4, 407, 1982.
256. Walker, C., Kristensen, F., Bettens, F., and De Weck, A. L., Lymphokine regulation of activated (G1) lymphocytes. I. Prostaglandin E-2 induced inhibition of interleukin 2 production, *J. Immunol.*, 130, 1770, 1983.
257. Chouaib, S., Chatenoud, L., Klatzmann, D., and Fradelizi, D., The mechanisms of inhibition of human IL2 production II. PGE2 induction of suppressor T lymphocytes, *J. Immunol.*, 132, 1851, 1984.
258. Naor, D., Suppressor cells: permitters and promotors of malignancy?, *Adv. Cancer Res.*, 29, 45, 1979.
259. Schultz, R. M., Pavilidis, N. A., Stylos, W. A., and Chirigos, M. A., Regulation of macrophage tumoricidal function: a role for prostaglandins of the E series, *Science*, 202, 320, 1978.
260. Taffett, S. M. and Russell, S. W., Macrophage-mediated tumor cell killing: regulation of expression of cytolytic activity by prostaglandin E, *J. Immunol.*, 126, 424, 1981.
261. Cheers, C., Pavlov, H., Riglar, C., and Madraso, E., Macrophage activation during experimental murine brucellosis. III. Do macrophages exert feedback control during brucellosis?, *Cell. Immunol.*, 49, 168, 1980.
262. Robinson, M. K., Truitt, G. A., Okayasu, T., and Wheelock, E. F., Enhanced suppressor macrophage activity associated with termination of the L5178Y cell tumor-dormant state in DBA/2 mice, *Cancer Res.*, 43, 5831, 1983.
263. Pollack, S., Micali, A., Kinne, D. W., Enker, W. L., Geller, N., Oettgen, H. F., and Hoffman, M. K., Endotoxin-induced in vitro release of interleukin-1 by cancer patients' monocytes: relation to stage of disease, *Int. J. Cancer*, 32, 733, 1983.
264. Zembala, M., Myttar, B., Ruggiero, I., Uracz, W., Popiela, T., and Czupryna, A., Suppressor cells and survival of patients with advanced gastric cancer, *J. Natl. Cancer Inst.*, 70, 233, 1983.
265. Lynch, N. R. and Salomon, J.-C., Tumour growth inhibition and potentiation of immunotherapy by indomethacin in mice, *J. Natl. Cancer Inst.*, 62, 117, 1979.
266. Fulton, A. M., In vivo effects of indomethacin on the growth of murine mammary tumors, *Cancer Res.*, 44, 2416, 1984.
267. Olsson, N. O., Caignard, A., Martin, M. S., and Martin, F., Effect of indomethacin on the growth of colon cancer cells in syngeneic rats, *Int. J. Immunopharmacol.*, 6, 329, 1984.

268. Djeu, J. Y., Heinbaugh, J. A., Holden, H. T., and Herberman, R. B., Role of macrophages in the augmentation of mouse natural killer cell activity by poly I:C and interferon, *J. Immunol.*, 122, 182, 1979.
269. Tracey, D. E., The requirement for macrophages in the augmentation of natural killer cell activity by BCG, *J. Immunol.*, 123, 840, 1979.
270. Tracey, D. E. and Adkinson, N. F., Prostaglandin synthesis inhibitors potentiate the BCG induced augmentation of natural killer cell activity, *J. Immunol.*, 125, 136, 1980.
271. Brunda, M. J., Taramelli, D., Holden, H. T., and Varesio, L., Suppression of in vitro maintenance and interferon-mediated augmentation of natural killer cell activity by adherent peritoneal cells from normal mice, *J. Immunol.*, 130, 1974, 1983.
272. Gerson, J. M., Varesio, L., and Herberman, R. B., Systemic and in situ natural killer and suppressor cell activities in mice bearing progressively growing murine sarcoma-virus induced tumors, *Int. J. Cancer*, 27, 243, 1981.
273. Polverini, P. J., Cotran, R. S., Gimbrone, M. A., Jr., and Unanue, E. R., Activated macrophages induce vascular proliferation, *Nature (London)*, 269, 804, 1977.
274. Martin, B. M., Gimbrone, M. A., Jr., Unanue, E. R., and Cotran, R. S., Stimulation of nonlymphoid mesenchymal cell proliferation by a macrophage-derived growth factor, *J. Immunol.*, 126, 1510, 1981.
275. Banda, M. J., Knighton, D. R., Hunt, T. K., and Werb, Z., Isolation of a nonmitogenic angiogenesis factor from wound fluid, *Proc. Natl. Acad. Sci. U.S.A.*, 79, 7773, 1982.
276. Polverini, P. J. and Leibovich, S. J., Induction of neovascularization in vivo and endothelial proliferation in vitro by tumor-associated macrophages, *Lab. Invest.*, 51, 635, 1984.
277. Roche, W. R., Mast cells and tumour angiogenesis: the tumor-mediated release of an endoethelial growth factor from mast cells, *Int. J. Cancer*, 36, 721, 1985.
278. Roche, W. R., The nature and significance of tumour-associated mast cells, *J. Pathol.*, 148, 175, 1986.
279. Starky, J. R., Liggitt, H. D., Jones, W., and Hosick, H. L., Influence of migratory blood cells on the attachment of tumor cells to vascular endothelium, *Int. J. Cancer*, 34, 535, 1984.
280. Terranova, V. P., Liotta, L. A., Russo, R. G., and Martin, G. R., Role of laminin in the attachment and metastasis of murine tumor cells, *Cancer Res.*, 42, 2265, 1982.
281. Perri, R. T., Vercellotti, G., McCarthy, J., Vessela, R. L., and Furcht, L. T., Laminin selectivity enhances monocyte-macrophage-mediated tumoricidal activity, *J. Lab. Clin. Med.*, 105, 30, 1985.
282. Raynor, R. H. and Reese, A. C., Effect of fibronectin on macrophage-induced tumor cell cytostasis, *Oncology*, 41, 420, 1984.
283. Martin, D. E., Reese, M., and Reese, A. C., Effect of plasma fibronectin, macrophages, and glycosaminoglycans on tumor cell growth, *Cancer Inv.*, 2, 339, 1984.
284. Schmidt, J. A., Nidel, S., Cohen, D., and Green, I., Interleukin 1, a potential regulator of fibroblast proliferation and collagen production, *J. Immunol.*, 128, 2177, 1982.
285. Dohlman, J. G., Payan, D. G., and Goetzl, E. J., Generation of a unique fibroblast-activating factor by human monocytes, *Immunology*, 52, 577, 1984.
286. Rickles, F. R. and Edwards, R. L., Activation of blood coagulation in cancer: trousseau's syndrome revisited, *Blood*, 62, 14, 1983.
287. Edwards, R. L. and Rickles, F. R., The role of monocyte tissue factor in the immune response, *Lymphokine Rep.*, 1, 181, 1980.
288. Geczy, C. L., The role of clotting processes in the action of lymphokines on macrophages, in *Lymphokines*, Vol. 8, Pick, E., Ed., Academic Press, New York, 1984, 201.
289. Inoue, Y., Geczy, C. L., Nelson, D. S., and Nelson, M., Lymphokine-like products of cultured tumour cells, *Immunology*, 48, 713, 1983.
290. Lorenzet, R., Peri, G., Locati, D., Allavena, P., Colucci, M., Semeraro, N., Mantovani, A., and Donati, M. B., Generation of procoagulant activity by monocular phagocytes: a possible mechanism contributing to blood clotting activation within malignant tissues, *Blood*, 62, 271, 1983.
291. Guarini, A., Acero, R., Alessio, G., Donati, M. B., Semeraro, N., and Mantovani, A., Procoagulant activity of macrophages associated with different murine neoplasms, *Int. J. Cancer*, 34, 581, 1984.
292. Gorelik, E., Bere, W. W., and Herberman, R. B., Role of NK cells in the antimetastatic effect of anticoagulant drugs, *Int. J. Cancer*, 33, 87, 1984.
293. Thomson, A. W., Moon, D. K., and Nelson, D. S., Unpublished observations.
294. Nelson, M. and Nelson, D. S., Unpublished observations.

Chapter 6

TUMOR-ASSOCIATED LEUKOCYTES IN METASTASIZING TUMORS

Alberto Mantovani, Barbara Bottazzi, Paola Allavena, and Claudia Balotta

TABLE OF CONTENTS

I. INTRODUCTION

Histopathologists have long recognized the presence of host leukocytic cells in the context or at the periphery of neoplastic tissues.[1-4] The biological and clinical significance of tumor-infiltrating inflammatory cells remains to a large extent obscure. Considerable efforts have been devoted to relate the degree and type of infiltrate determined by classical histopathology to prognosis, but conflicting results have been reported and firm conclusions are difficult to draw.[1-4] The application of more accurate methods to quantitate tumor-associated leukocytes may shed new light on this area as indicated by the striking and intriguing prognostic significance of eosinophils in colon cancer.[5] The availability of monoclonal antibody (moab) defined markers of leukocyte subpopulations offers an approach to investigate the presence and significance of defined subsets of inflammatory cells in neoplastic tissues.

While more precise and quantitative identification of tumor-associated leukocytes may solve unsettled issues related to the histopathology of inflammatory cells in neoplasms, the availaiblity of techniques to purify cells of the lymphoreticular infiltrate and to probe their function has considerably improved our understanding of the complexity of functions which can be mediated by *in situ* leukocytes. Information concerning the functional properties of tumor-infiltrating leukocytes is relatively abundant, though incomplete, in rodent systems, whereas functional data on human neoplasms are scanty and fragmentary and confined to a few tumor types. Previous reviews on the histopathology of tumor-infiltrating leukocytes[1-4] and on tumor-associated macrophages and NK cells[6-8] provide the background and framework for the present chapter that will center upon the origin and functional properties of inflammatory cells associated with metastatic tumors of rodents and, to the extent that is possible, humans.

II. TUMOR-ASSOCIATED MACROPHAGES

A. Origin and Regulation of Accumulation in Primary and Metastatic Tumors

Rodent and human tumors vary widely in their macrophage infiltrate.[6,7] The percentage of tumor-associated macrophages (TAM) of each individual tumor is usually maintained as a stable property upon transplantation.[9,10] A decrease in the frequency of TAM is sometimes observed during the final stages of tumor growth in rodents,[6,7,10] presumably because of exhaustion of the bone marrow capacity to supply adequate numbers of precursors.

The maintainance of constant levels of TAM in a growing neoplastic tissue is at least partially dependent upon the recruitment of circulating monocytic precursors[11-13] but there is also evidence that TAM may to some extent proliferate *in situ*.[11,14,15] No quantitative estimate of the relative contribution to accumulation of TAM of recruitment from circulating monocytes vs. *in situ* proliferation is presently available.

The mechanisms determining the amount of macrophages infiltrating tumors have not been completely elucidated. Early studies showed a correlation between immunogenicity and levels of TAM in rat neoplasms with different propensity to metastasize.[16,17] Moreover, with some tumors transplantation into nude or thymus-deprived animals with defective specific immunity resulted in neoplastic tissues less infiltrated by macrophages.[16] These findings would suggest that the entry of blood monocytes into tumors and/or their *in situ* proliferation is mainly dependent on specific antitumor immune responses. Subsequent studies in mouse tumors did not support the general validity of this conclusion. Evans and co-workers,[18,19] and Talmadge and co-workers[20] in two large series of mouse tumors found no correlation between immunogenicity and macrophage levels *in situ*. Moreover transplantation in mice with defective specific immunity (thymectomized or node or UV-irradiated) did not affect the accumulation of TAM in various murine sarcomas.[19-21] Collectively, the available evidence suggests that specific immunity is not the sole or major determinant of the number of macrophages accumulating in neoplastic tissues, although it may play a role in some models.

The importance attributed to mechanisms of natural resistance in surveillance[22] and control of tumor dissemination[22-26] together with the recognition that NK cells secrete inflammatory lymphokines[27-29] lead us to investigate whether NK activity is an important determinant of macrophage accumulation into tumors. We transplanted three mouse metastatic neoplasms into mice with congenital (beige) or induced (anti-asialo GM1) deficiency of NK activity and found no substantial change in the levels of TAM.[30] These results suggest that NK cell-mediated resistance does not play an appreciable role in the regulation of levels of TAM. However a contribution of NK cells to infiltration of nascent tumors or a role of natural effectors other than NK[31] cannot be excluded on the basis of these data.

Products of neoplastic cells may play a pivotal role in regulating the entry of mononuclear phagocytes in neoplastic tissues. Impairment of the responsiveness of mononuclear phagocytes to chemoattractants and defective in vivo inflammatory responses have been demonstrated in tumor bearing animals and humans.[32-36] Defective systemic chemotaxis of monocytes in tumor-bearing hosts may be related to a soluble inhibitor[37,38] and the retroviral immunosuppressive protein P15E has been implicated in this defect.[39,40]

While results on chemotaxis inhibitors point to interference with monocyte entry as a means of subverting host resistance, along a different line various tumor cells of human or murine origin have been shown to release products with chemotactic activity for monocytes.[41-45] A tumor-derived chemotactic factor (TDCF) has been described as a glycoprotein of 12000 mol wt found in the supernatant of neoplastic cells and, in lesser amounts, of some normal cell lines.[44,46] TDCF is chemotactic for monocytes in a Boyden chamber assay but does not affect the migration of lymphocytes, polymorphs, and endothelial cells.[44,47,134] In a series of 11 murine tumors, heterogeneous in terms of origin, histology, and transplantation history, some correlation was found between percentage of TAM in growing tumors and amounts of TDCF produced in vitro.[43] In this study variants with different metastatic capacity did not differ for TDCF production. Release of chemoattractant was also found with human tumor lines and freshly isolated ovarian carcinoma cells with similar physico-chemical and biological properties.[44,45] In a series of 24 patients with ovarian carcinoma a significant, though far from strict, correlation was found between the percentage of TAM and the amounts of TDCF activity released by tumor cells.[45] These results are compatible with the hypothesis that production of chemoattractants by tumor cells plays a role in the regulation of the macrophage infiltrate of neoplasms. It is of interest in this light, that platelet-derived growth factor (PDGF) is chemotactic in vitro for monocytes, thus raising the interesting possibility that growth factors involved in malignant transformation may be involved in recruiting mononuclear phagocytes at the tumor site.

The relationship between number of TAM and propensity to metastasize has been the object of conflicting reports. Early reports with rat tumors, suggested that less infiltrated neoplasms were more metastatic.[16,17] In contrast, studies with mouse sarcoma and melanoma lines failed to evidentiate any correlation between metastatic potential and levels of TAM.[20] In our early studies with two lines of a murine sarcoma, the metastatic tumor was less infiltrated than the nonmetastatic one.[48] However, when the analysis was extended to a series of sublines with different metastatic potential derived from the same sarcoma, the correlation was not confirmed, as was also the case with sublines from Rous sarcoma virus-induced tumors.[134] In murine mammary carcinomas, no correlation was found between macrophage content and propensity to spontaneously seed at distant anatomical sites or to colonize lungs upon i.v., inoculation,[49-52] although in one study macrophages infiltrating metastatic tumors were different in terms of size, distribution, and function compared to those associated with nonmetastatic carcinomas.[50,51]

The infiltration of macrophage into metastatic foci has been the object of less extensive studies.[49,53-55] Individual established metastases of murine sarcoma and of B16 melanoma had different levels of TAM. However, when pooled data of established secondary foci were considered[54,55] or when pooled metastases were analyzed,[49,53] no appreciable difference in macrophage content was found between secondary deposits and primary lesions. While these studies refer to established macroscopic metastasis, limited information is available on the macrophage infiltrate at the early steps of implantation and growth of secondaries. Bugelski et al.[55] recently reported a detailed analysis of the early macrophage infiltrate of B16 melanoma lung colonies obtained by injecting tumor cells intravenously. The macrophage content of small B16 secondaries (<700 cells) was much greater than that of larger lesions. In this study tumor cells were injected intravenously, a route of administration associated with early transient hematological alterations not found under conditions of spontaneous dissemination. If these differences are uninfluencial and the greater macrophage infiltrate of early lesions is also found in natural secondaries from this and other tumors, these results may explain the differential modulation of primary tumor growth and metastasis by macrophage toxins which inhibit the former and enhance the early steps of the latter.[12,56-58]

B. Functional Properties of TAM and Regulation of Metastasis

Selected aspects of the functional status of TAM (e.g., tumoricidal activity) have been the object of rather extensive studies, but even on these, information on macrophages in primary tumors with metastatic potential or secondary deposits is scanty and fragmentary. Macrophages can act as accessory cells by presenting antigen in the context of class II major histocompatibility gene (Ia) products and by providing a proliferative and differentiation signal with IL-1.[59] We are not aware of published reports on Ia antigen expression and IL-1 secretion by TAM. Our group has recently examined TAM from a series of murine sarcomas including two metastatic tumors. TAM had a considerably higher frequency of Ia⁺ cells than peritoneal macrophages with values ranging from 20 to 70%. Upon culture expression of Ia declined but, exposure to lymphokine supernatants (presumably interferon-γ) maintained and augmented the frequency of Ia⁺ cells. TAM acted as antigen presenting cells in a secondary in vitro response to GAT. The reasons for the higher expression of Ia in TAM compared to resident macrophages are unclear. An important role of specific antitumor immunity is suggested by preliminary data showing lesser Ia expression in TAM from one tumor transplanted into nude mice.

The function of TAM which has been most extensively studied is tumor cytotoxicity.[60,61] In general, TAM from progressively growing malignant tumors were not found activated for tumor cytotoxicity,[6,7,48,52,53] with some exceptions. In particular, Loveless and Heppner[50] reported that TAM from metastatic mammary carcinomas were more frequently cytotoxic than cells isolated from nonmetastatic tumors. Only two studies investigated the cytotoxic potential of macrophages isolated from secondary deposits.[53,54] TAM from pulmonary metastases were not activated for tumor cytotoxicity, but in vitro exposure to free or lyposome-encapsulated stimuli augmented the cytotocidal capacity of these cells.[53,54] In two studies with rodent metastatic tumors[52,53] and in human ovarian cancer (see below) intratumor macrophages exposed to activating agents (e.g. endotoxin) developed lower levels of tumoricidal activity than inflammatory macrophages. There were two groups who reported that the multistep process of metastasis was not associated with the appearance of variant tumor cells in secondary foci resistant to macrophage-mediated killing.[52,53,62] In other murine tumors augmentation of resistance to cytotoxicity has been associated with neoplastic progression.[52,58,63,64] Differences in the in vitro end points used to assess macrophage killing[65] and/or in the intrinsic properties of the tumors examined may explain this apparent discrepancy.

Macrophages can kill antibody-sensitized tumor cells and TAM are potent effectors of this reactivity.[6,65-68] We are not aware of data on the ADCC effector potential of cells infiltrating metastatic foci.

Mononuclear phagocytes are capable of producing growth factors such as IL-1 and PDGF-like substances.[69] It is therefore not surprising that these cells can promote the growth in vitro of tumor cells. Macrophages isolated from various murine sarcomas and carcinomas and human ovarian carcinoma have been shown to enhance the proliferative capacity of tumor cells.[6,7,48,52,66,70-78] The growth promoting capacity of TAM was usually better observed at low effector to target cell ratios or with tumor cells in suboptimal culture conditions. The mechanisms by which mononuclear phagocytes, and TAM in particular, can enhance tumor cell proliferation in vitro have not been elucidated, though it appears likely that the above-mentioned macrophage-derived growth factors are involved in this reactivity.

Although the direct interaction of macrophages with tumor cells resulting either in killing or growth promotion has been the aspect of the biology of TAM most extensively investigated, other properties of mononuclear phagocytes for which little or nor information is available may have an equal or greater importance in vivo. Thus TAM from some, but not all, murine tumors have been shown to produce increased amounts of procoagulant activity (PCA).[79,80] The reasons for enhanced PCA in TAM are not clear, but recent evidence indicates that selected tumor lines may act directly on monocytes, triggering synthesis of PCA.[81] It is conceivable that macrophage PCA may contribute to fibrin deposition in neoplastic tissues,[82,83] thus affecting the motility of tumor cells, the entry of other effector cells and angiogenesis.

Upon membrane perturbation or phagocytosis mononuclear phagocytes produce reactive oxygen intermediates (ROI) which can play a role in the microbicidal and tumoricidal capacity of macrophages.[84] ROI produced by phagocytes can be mutagenic[85,86] and TAM from murine mammary carcinomas have been reported to release mutagenic activity.[87] One could therefore speculate that TAM may contribute to generation of diversity within neoplasms, though direct proof of this is missing.

Cells of the monocyte-macrophage lineage are potent producers of proteinases. We have recently found that TAM from various murine sarcomas have increase amounts of the neutral serine protease plasminogen activator, thus resembling thioglicollate elicited peritoneal macrophages.[135] Therefore one might infer that macrophage-derived proteases may contribute to tissue invasion by tumor cells. Along the same line it has been reported that macrophage-derived soluble factors induce collagenolytic activity in Lewis lung carcinoma cells.[88]

The formation of new blood vessels is a crucial step in the growth of neoplastic tissues[89] and provides the necessary conditions for dissemination at distant anatomical sties. Tumor-infiltrating macrophages are likely to affect the induction of neovascularization and the function of blood vessels. Macrophage products, IL-1 in particular, have been shown to modulate crucial functions of vessel wall cells, such as PCA, production of platelet-activating factor (PAF) and arachidonate metabolism.[90] Moreover, TAM, by favoring fibrin deposition via PCA production,[79,80] may indirectly promote new vessel formation. Inflammatory macrophages have been shown to induce neovascularization of corneal tissues[91] and more recently TAM from a rat tumor have been shown to have angiogenic activity.[92]

The information on functions of TAM in metastatic tumors and their secondary deposits discussed so far refers to murine neoplasms. Comparatively, little information is available on TAM in human tumors. The functional status of peripheral blood monocytes is not necessarily representative of that of tumor-infiltrating macrophages.[66,70,71,93,99] Thus in breast carcinoma considerable differences were found in lysozyme content in peripheral vs. tumor-associated macrophages.[96] Along the same line macrophages from bronchoalveolar spaces of tumor-bearing lungs had defective Fc-receptor function.[95] A considerable amount of data has accumulated on macrophages in pleural or peritoneal effusions, in particular from carcinomas of the ovary.[66,67,70,71,93,94,98-100] Although effusions have been utilized as a convenient tool to characterize inflammatory cells from an anatomical site directly involved in neoplasia, it is now clear that macrophages associated with ascites can differ in several respects from those associated with solid tumors.[67,93,94] For instance, from a cytochemical point of view, higher numbers of ascites macrophages are peroxidase-positive compared to TAM from solid ovarian carcinoma. Solid ovarian cancer TAM are relatively more refractory to activation for tumor cytotoxicity than peritoneal effectors, as found in some murine tumors,[52,53] though with considerable inter-individual variability among different patients.[93] As already mentioned TAM from ascitic or solid tumors of the ovary have also been shown to have the potential to promote tumor growth in vitro.[66,70,71]

Tumor cell properties may play a crucial role in determining the outcome of the interaction with leukocytes and considerable heterogeneity in antigen expression or susceptibility to effector mechanisms including autologous intratumor macrophages has been found.[70,71,93,94] The regulation of tumor cell susceptibility to effector mechanisms in metastatic foci may represent an important point for the development of successful therapeutic approaches based on immunity. It is of interest in this perspective that certain cancer chemotherapy agents can modulate the susceptibility of target cells to killing mediated by mononuclear phagocytes.[101]

C. In Vivo Role of TAM in the Control of Metastasis

The complexity and diverse significance of in vitro measured functional properties of TAM discussed in the previous paragraph caution against simplistic extrapolations from in vitro activities to in vivo role. The question of the in vivo relevance of TAM in the regulation of metastasis has been approached by administering compounds that inhibit macrophage functions, by adoptively transfering macrophages, and by correlating in vitro interactions with metastatic potential. The available, to some extent conflicting evidence on the last point was already discussed in the previous paragraph.

The administration to tumor-bearing mice of macrophage toxins, such as silica and carrageenan, resulted in augmentation of metastasis in various tumor models.[56,57] The specificity of these agents administered in vivo for cells of the monocyte-macrophage lineage is questionable, but indirect evidence suggested that effects of these poisons on T-cells, NK cells, and tumor cells themselves were not involved in augmentation of metastasis. Similarly, glucocorticoid hormones enhance metastasis in experimental[12] and possibly human[102,103] neoplasia, and interference with TAM, which were indeed decreased in hydrocortisone treated mice, was suggested to play major role in these effects.[12] Interestingly enough, macrophage toxins and glucocorticoid hormones concomitantly decreased the growth of the primary tumors.[12,56,58] The augmentation of metastasis by these compounds depended upon their effects on the early steps of implantation and growth in secondary foci. The subsequent growth of established secondaries was actually decreased as was the case for subcutaneously growing tumors.[12] These results were interpreted to indicate that, in the tumors examined, TAM were providing the optimal conditions for neoplastic growth, by secretion growth factors and by directly or indirectly (via procoagulant activity) favoring angiogenesis; however, the mononuclear phagocyte system acted as a mechanism of restraint of some early step of implantation and growth at distant sites. The divergent roles of mononuclear phagocytes in the regulation of growth of primary tumors and early steps of metastasis could be explained by the recent observations of Bugelski et al.[55] who found much higher macrophage infiltrate in very early secondary foci (see also the previous paragraph for discussion). These conditions of high macrophage: tumor cell ratio would permit the expression of tumoricidal activity and mononuclear phagocytes would inhibit the early phases of implantation and growth at secondary foci.

Adoptive transfer has been utilized as an approach to directly evaluate the role of macrophages in the regulation of tumor growth and metastasis. Transplantation of tumor cells mixed with macrophages in normal or monocytopenic hosts has resulted in earlier appearance or faster growth of various murine tumors.[12,73-75,77,78] These results, together with the functional data on TAM discussed above, support the concept that macrophages in some tumors and at some steps of pregression, may provide the conditions for optimal neoplastic proliferation, directly by producing growth factors or indirectly, via for instance induction of vascularization.

Macrophages have also been transferred intravenously in an effort to directly study their role in the control of metastasis. Transfer of macrophages activated for tumor cytotoxicity has resulted in inhibition of lung colonization.[104,105] These results, together with the effect of in vivo activation of macrophages which is discussed elsewhere in this book, support the concept that macrophages, once activated for tumor cytotoxicity, can restrain metastasis[62] While macrophages rendered tumoricidal may restrain metastasis, by directly killing tumor cells or by recruiting other effectors, it has been shown that thiogliocollate-elicited macrophages inoculated intravenously enhance the formation of lung colonies.[78,106,107] This activity is unique to peritoneal macrophages elicited by Brewer's thioglicollate medium and not found in resident macrophages or macrophages elicited by other inflammatory agents.[107] Augmentation of metastasis by thioglicollate-elicited macrophages has been related to inhibition of NK activity[106] and the induction of intravascular reactions.[107] Macrophages represent a tissue phase in the natural history of mononuclear phagocytes and do not circulate in blood under normal conditions. This consideration, together with the profound effects of these cells on hemostatic mechanisms, cautions against "mechanical" extrapolation of results obtained by i.v. inoculation of elicited macrophages to physiological conditions. Mouse strains with selective defects of macrophage tumoricidal activity have been carefully characterized[108] and they may represent an important experimental system to investigate the role of macrophage killing in the control of primary tumors and metastasis. Work along this line is currently in progress in this laboratory.

III. TUMOR-ASSOCIATED LYMPHOID CELLS

Little, if any, information is available concerning the functional properties of lymphoid cells associated with secondary foci, with the notable exception of pleural and peritoneal effusions. Therefore the present discussion will deal with selected aspects of the biology of tumor-associated lymphoid cells (TAL) from neoplasms with metastatic capacity, rather than with TAL from metastases. NK activity have been suggested to play an important role in the control of metastasis, as reviewed elsewhere in this book, and has been analyzed in TAL from murine and human tumors.[8] TAL from malignant human tumors usually have low or negligible levels of NK activity. With appreciable frequency, solid nasopharyngeal carcinoma, ovarian carcinomas, and effusion fluids yielded lymphoid cells with detectable NK activity, though low compared with blood lymphocytes.[8,109-112] In ovarian cancer, NK activity was higher and more frequently detectable in peritoneal effusions compared with solid lesions. This observation may reflect a greater accessibility of the serosal compartment to NK effectors compared with solid tissues.

Multiple factors are probably involved in the defective NK cytotoxicity of lymphoid cells *in situ*. Cell-mediated suppression of NK activity has been demonstrated, and *in situ* phagocytic cells have been shown to interfere with NK cell function, although in some patients lymphocytic suppressor were found.[110,113-115] NK cells, identified morphologically or with monoclonal antibodies in tissue sections or disaggregated specimens, have been shown by various investigators to be represented in low frequency in TAL.[8,116-119] In apparent discrepancy with these results Moy et al.[120] recently reported high percentages of cells bearing monoclonal antibody-defined surface markers of NK, with defective function, in lung cancer. The poor localization of NK cells in most established metastatic tumors is intriguing. In allografts, NK cells are present initially in large numbers but disappear thereafter.[121] It would be important to have accurate information on very early primary or secondary malignant lesions, but this data is lacking at present. In general, little is known concerning the relationship between the blood and tissue compartment for NK cells. A recently described in vitro assay for the migration of LGL/NK cells may help to elucidate some aspects of the extravasation of NK cells.[122]

A crucial question concerning the lymphoid infiltrate of tumors is whether it contains lymphocytic effectors which specifically recognize and kill autologous neoplastic cells. In ^{51}Cr release assyas, 20 to 30% of the patients with a variety of cancers have blood lymphocytes cytotoxic against freshly isolated autologous tumor cells. Autologous tumor killing was detected in nasopharingeal, lung, breast, and colon carcinoma, and in mesenchymal tumors, whereas reactivity was observed rarely or not at all in oat cell carcinoma of the lung and in ovarian carcinoma.[123-127] Relevant to the present discussion on metastasis is the finding that the presence of lymphocyte-mediate cytotoxicity was associated with better prognosis in sarcomas and lung carcinomas,[128,129] whereas such association was not found in colon cancer.[130] Even in those patients who had lymphocytes reactive against the autologous tumor in peripheral blood, TAL were unreactive.[123-130] A recent report suggests that TAL, though lacking cytotoxicity against autologous tumor cells, contain precursors capable of killing after culture with Il-2 at a higher frequency than blood lymphocytes.[131] These observations would suggest that cytotoxic precursors do localize at the tumor site but fail to express cytotoxic capacity *in situ*. The occurrence of macrophage and lymphoid cell-mediated suppressor mechanisms has been reported in *in situ* inflammatory cells[132,133] and may account for these findings.

IV. CONCLUDING REMARKS

The occurrence of leukocytes in the context of neoplastic tissues has long been recognized, but several aspects of their origin, regulation, and function remain to be elucidated. Attention has focused largely on the direct interactions occurring between leukocytes and tumor cells and therefore the cytotoxic activity of tumor-associated inflammatory cells has been emphasized and analyzed in some detail. However the information now available suggests that functions of *in situ* leukocytes other than tumor cell killing may be as important in the biology of neoplastic tissues. Among these, the production of growth factors, the interaction with hemostatic mechanisms, the release of mutagenic ROI and neutral proteases and the capacity to induce angiogenesis have the potential to play important roles at some stages of neoplastic progression and metastasis. The complexity of functions that leukocytes can mediate and their ambivalence in the tumor-host relationship defies any simplistic view of the significance of tumor-associated inflammatory cells. Since successful modulation of host resistance in neoplastic disorders will ultimately depending upon changing the tumor-host relationship at the tumor site, better understanding of the regulation and function of tumor-associated leukocytes may prove valuable for application of immunomodulation to metastatic neoplasia, by providing a less empirical basis for planning, explanations for failures and, possibly success.

ACKNOWLEDGMENTS

This work was suppported by grant ROI CA 26824 from the National Cancer Institute, USA and Contract No. 84.00656.44 (special project Oncology) from CNR, Roma, Italy. The generous support of the Italian Association for Cancer Research is gratefully acknowledged.

REFERENCES

1. Underwood, J. C., Lymphoreticular infiltration in human tumours: prognostic and biological implications: a review, *Br. J. Cancer,* 30, 538, 1974.
2. Ioachim, H. L., The stromal reaction of tumors: an expression of immune surveillance, *J. Natl. Cancer Inst.,* 57, 465, 1976.
3. Kreider, J. W., Barlett, G. L., and Butkiewicz, B. L., Relationship of tumor leukocytic infiltration to host defense mechanisms and prognosis, *Cancer Met. Rev.,* 3, 53, 1984.
4. Haskill, S., *Ed., Tumor Immunity in Prognosis. The Role of Mononuclear Cell Infiltration,* Marcel Dekker, New York, 1982.
5. Pretlow, T. P., Keith, E. F., Cryar, A. K., Bartolucci, A. A., Pitts, A. M., Pretlow, T. G. II, Kimball, P. M., and Boohaker, E. A., Eosinophil infiltration of human colonic carcinomas as a prognostic indicator, *Cancer Res.,* 43, 2997, 1983.
6. Evans, R. and Haskill, S., Activities of macrophages within and peripheral to the tumor mass, in *The Reticuloendothelial System, a Comprehensive Treatise,* Vol. 5, Herberman, R. B., Ed., Plenum Press, New York, 1983, 155.
7. Mantovani, A., Origin and function of tumor-associated macrophages in murine and human neoplasms, in *Progress in Immunology,* Vol. 5, Yamamura, Y. and Tada, T., Eds., Academic Press, Orlando, Fla., 1983, 1001.
8. Introna, M. and Mantovani, A., Natural killer cells in human solid tumors, *Cancer Met. Rev.,* 2, 237, 1983.
9. Evans, R., Macrophages and neoplasms: new insight and their implication in tumor immunobiology, *Cancer Met. Rev.,* 1, 227, 1982.
10. Evans, R., Macrophages in syngeneic animal tumours, *Transplantation,* 14, 468, 1972.
11. Evans, R. and Cullen, R. T., In situ proliferation of intratumor macrophages, *J. Leukocyte Biol.,* 35, 561, 1984.
12. Acero, R., Polentarutti, N., Bottazzi, B., Alberti, S., Ricci, M. R., Bizzi, A., and Mantovani, A., Effect of hydrocortisone on the macrophage content, growth and metastasis of transplanted murine tumors, *Int. J. Cancer,* 33, 95, 1984.
13. Kaizer, L. and Lala, P. K., Post-mitotic age of mononuclear cells migrating into Ta-3(St) solid tumors, *Cell Tissue Kinet.,* 10, 279, 1977.
14. Stewart, C. C. and Beetham, K. L., Cytocidal activity and proliferative ability of macrophages infiltrating the EMT6 tumor, *Int. J. Cancer,* 22, 152, 1978.
15. Stewart, C. C., Local proliferation of mononuclear phagocytes in tumors, *J. Reticuloendothel. Soc.,* 34, 23, 1983.
16. Eccles, S. A. and Alexander, P., Macrophage content of tumours in relation to metastatic spread and host immune reaction, *Nature (London),* 250, 667, 1974.
17. Moore, K. and Moore, M., Intra-tumour host cells of transplanted rat neoplasms of different immunogenicity, *Int. J. Cancer,* 19, 803, 1977.
18. Evans, R. and Lawler, E. M., Macrophage content and immunogenicity of C57BL/6J and BALB/cByJ methylcholanthrene-induced sarcomas, *Int. J. Cancer,* 26, 831, 1980.

19. Evans, R. and Eidlen, D. M., Macrophage accumulation in transplanted tumors is not dependent on host immune responsiveness or presence of tumor-associated rejection antigens, *J. Reticuloendothel. Soc.*, 30, 425, 1981.

20. Talmadge, J. E., Key, M., and Fidler, I. J., Macrophage content of metastatic and nonmetastatic rodent neoplasms, *J. Immunol.*, 126, 2245, 1981.

21. Szymaniec, S. and James, K., Studies on the Fc receptor bearing cells in a transplanted methylcholanthrene induced mouse fibrosarcoma, *Br. J. Cancer*, 33, 36, 1976.

22. Herberman, R. B. and Ortaldo, J. R., Natural killer cells: their role in defenses against disease, *Science*, 214, 24, 1981.

23. Talmadge, J. E., Meyers, K. M., Prieur, D. J., and Starkey, J. R., Role of NK cells in tumour growth and metastasis in beige mice, *Nature (London)*, 284, 622, 1980.

24. Hanna, N. and Fidler, I. J., Role of natural killer cells in the destruction of circulating tumor emboli, *J. Natl. Cancer Inst.*, 65, 801, 1980.

25. Hanna, N. and Fidler, I. J., Relationship between metastatic potential and resistance to natural killer cell-mediated cytotoxicity in three murine tumor systems, *J. Natl. Cancer Inst.*, 66, 1183, 1981.

26. Gorelik, E., Wiltrout, R. H., Okumura, K., Habu, S., and Herberman, R. B., Role of NK cells in the control of metastatic spread and growth of tumor cells in mice, *Int. J. Cancer*, 30, 107, 1982.

27. Kasahara, T., Djeu, J. Y., Dougherthy, S. F., and Oppenheim, J. J., Capacity of human large granular lymphocytes (LGL) to produce multiple lymphokines: interleukin 2, interferon, and colony stimulating factor, *J. Immunol.*, 131, 2379, 1983.

28. Sauder, D. N., Mounessa, N. L., Katz, S. I., Dinarello, C. A., and Gallin, J. I., Chemotactic cytokines: the role of leukocytic pyrogen and epidermal cell thymocyte-activating factor in neutrophil chemotaxis, *J. Immunol.*, 132, 828, 1984.

29. Scala, G., Allavena, P., Djeu, J. Y., Kasahara, T., Ortaldo, J. R., Herberman, R. B., and Oppenheim, J. J., Human large granular lymphocytes (IGL) are potent producers of interleukin 1, *Nature (London)*, 309, 56, 1984.

30. Polentarutti, N., Acero, R., Bottazzi, B., Taraboletti, G., and Mantovani, A., The macrophage content of tumors is unrelated to levels of NK cell-mediated resistance, *J. Leukocyte Biol.*, in press.

31. Stutman, O. and Cuttito, M. J., Normal levels of natural cytotoxic cells against solid tumours in NK-deficient beige mice, *Nature (London)*, 290, 254, 1981.

32. Boetcher, D. A. and Leonard, E. J., Abnormal monocyte chemotactic response in cancer patients, *J. Natl. Cancer Inst.*, 52, 1091, 1974.

33. Normann, S. J., Schardt, M., and Sorkin, E., Biphasic depression of macrophage function after tumor transplantation, *Int. J. Cancer*, 28, 185, 1981.

34. Normann, S. J. and Sorkin, E., Cell-specific defect in monocyte function during tumor growth, *J. Natl. Cancer Inst.*, 57, 135, 1976.

35. Normann, S. J. and Sorkin, E., Inhibition of macrophage chemotaxis by neoplastic and other rapidly proliferating cells in vitro, *Cancer Res.*, 37, 705, 1977.

36. Stevenson, M. M. and Meltzer, M. S., Depressed chemotactic responses in vitro peritoneal macrophages from tumor-bearing mice, *J. Natl. Cancer Inst.*, 57, 847, 1976.

37. Snyderman, R. and Pike, M. C., An inhibitor of macrophage chemotaxis produced by neoplasms, *Science*, 192, 370, 1976.

38. Snyderman, R., Pike, M. C., and Cianciolo, G. J., An inhibitor of macrophage accumulation produced by neoplasms: its role in abrogating host resistance to cancer, in *Mononuclear Phagocytes*, van Furth, R., Ed., Martinus Nijhoff, Hingham, Mass., 1980, 569.

39. Cianciolo, G. J., Hunter, J., Silva, J., Haskill, J. S., and Snyderman, R., Inhibitors of monocyte responses to chemotaxins are present in human cancerous effusion and react with monoclonal antibodies to the P15(E) structural protein of retroviruses, *J. Clin. Invest.*, 68, 831, 1981.

40. Snyderman, R. and Cianciolo, G. J., Immunosuppressive activity of the retroviral envelope protein P15E and its possible relationship to neoplasia, *Immunol. Today*, 5, 240, 1984.

41. Lane, R. D., Kaplan, A. M., Snodgrass, M. J., and Szakal, A. K., Characterization of a macrophage chemokinetic factor in tumor cell culture media, *J. Reticuloendothel. Soc.*, 31, 171, 1982.

42. Meltzer, M. S., Stevenson, M. M., and Leonard, E. J., Characterization of macrophage chemotaxins in tumor cell cultures and comparison with lymphocyte-derived chemotactic factors, *Cancer Res.*, 37, 721, 1977.

43. Bottazzi, B., Polentarutti, N., Acero, R., Balsari, A., Boraschi, D., Ghezzi, P., Salmona, M., and Mantovani, A., Regulation of the macrophage content of neoplasms by chemoattractants, *Science*, 220, 210, 1983.

44. Bottazzi, B., Polentarutti, N., Balsari, A., Boraschi, D., Ghezzi, P., Salmona, M., and Mantovani, A., Chemotactic activity for mononuclear phagocytes of culture supernatants from murine and human tumor cells: evidence for a role in the regulation of the macrophage content of neoplastic tissues, *Int. J. Cancer*, 31, 55, 1983.

45. Bottazzi, B., Ghezzi, P., Taraboletti, G., Salmona, M., Colombo, N., Bonazzi, C., Mangioni, C., and Mantovani, A., Tumor-derived chemotactic factor(s) from human ovarian carcinoma: evidence for a role in the regulation of the macrophage content of the neoplastic tissues, *Int. J. Cancer*, in press.

46. Valente, A. J., Fowler, S. R., Sprague, E. A., Kelley, J. L., Suenram, A. C., and Schwartz, C. J., Initial characterization of a peripheral blood mononuclear cell chemoattractant derived from cultured arterial smooth muscle cells, *Am. J. Pathol.*, 117, 409, 1984.

47. Dejana, E., Languino, L. R., Polentarutti, N., Balconi, G., Rykewaert, J. J., Larrieu, M. J., Donati, M. B., Mantovani, A., and Marguerie, G., Interaction between fibrinogen and cultured endothelial cells. Induction of migration and specific binding, *J. Clin. Invest.*, 75, 11, 1985.

48. Mantovani, A., Effects on in vitro tumor growth of murine macrophages isolated from sarcoma lines differing in immunogenicity and metastasizing capacity, *Int. J. Cancer*, 22, 741, 1978.

49. Nash, J. R. G., Price, J. E., and Tarin, D., Macrophage content and colony-forming potential in mouse mammary carcinomas, *Br. J. Cancer*, 43, 478, 1981.

50. Loveless, S. E. and Heppner, G. H., Tumor-associated macrophages in mouse of mammary tumors. I. Differential cytotoxicity of macrophages from metastatic and nonmetastatic tumors, *J. Immunol.*, 131, 2074, 1983.

51. Mahoney, K. H., Fulton, A. M., and Heppner, G. H., Tumor-associated macrophages of mouse mammary tumors. II. Differential distribution of macrophages metastatic and nonmetastatic tumors, *J. Immunol.*, 131, 2079, 1983.

52. North, S. M. and Nicolson, G. L., Heterogeneity in the sensitivities of the 13762NF rat mammary adenocarcinoma cell clones to cytolysis mediated by extra- and intratumoral macrophages, *Cancer Res.*, 45, 1453, 1985.

53. Mantovani, A., In vitro effects on tumor cells of macrophages isolated from an early-passage chemically-induced murine sarcoma and from its spontaneous metastases, *Int. J. Cancer*, 27, 221, 1981.

54. Key, M. E., Macrophages in cancer metastases and their relevance to metastatic growth, *Cancer Metastasis Rev.*, 2, 75, 1983.

55. Bugelski, P. J., Kirsh, R. L., Sowinski, J. M., and Poste, G., Changes in the macrophage content of lung metastases at different stages in tumor growth, *Am. J. Pathol.*, 118, 419, 1985.

56. Mantovani, A., Giavazzi, R., Polentarutti, N., Spreafico, F., and Garattini, S., Divergent effects of macrophage toxins on growth of primary tumors and lung metastases in mice, *Int. J. Cancer*, 25, 617, 1980.

57. Sadler, T. E., Jones, P. D. E., and Castro, J. E., The effects of altered phagocytic activity on growth of primary and metastatic tumor, in *The Macrophage and Cancer*, James, K., McBride, B., and Stuart, A., Eds., Econoprint, Edinburgh, 1977, 155.

58. Yamamura, Y., Fischer, B. C., Harnaha, J. B., and Proctor, J. W., Heterogeneity of murine mammary adenocarcinoma cell subpopulations. In vitro and in vivo resistance to macrophage cytotoxicity and its association with metastatic capacity, *Int. J. Cancer*, 33, 67, 1984.

59. Unanue, E. R., Beller, D. I., Lu, C. Y., and Allen, P. M., Antigen presentation: comments on its regulation and mechanism, *J. Immunol.*, 132, 1, 1984.

60. Adams, D. O. and Snyderman, R., Do macrophages destroy nascent tumors?, *J. Natl. Cancer Inst.*, 62, 1341, 1979.

61. Hibbs, J. B., The macrophage as a tumoricidal effector cell: a review of in vitro and in vivo studies on the mechanism of the activated macrophage nonspecific cytotoxic reaction, in *The Macrophage in Neoplasia*, Fink, M. A., Ed., Academic Press, New York, 1976, 83.

62. Fidler, I. J. and Poste, G., Macrophage-mediated destruction of malignant tumor cells and new strategies for the therapy of metastatic disease, *Springer Semin. Immunopathol.*, 5, 161, 1982.

63. Miner, K. M. and Nicolson, G. L., Differences in the sensitivities of murine metastatic lymphoma/lymphosarcoma variants to macrophage-mediated cytolysis and/or cytostatic, *Cancer Res.*, 43, 2063, 1983.

64. Urban, J. L. and Schreiber, H., Selection of macrophage-resistant progressor tumor variants by the normal host, *J. Exp. Med.*, 157, 642, 1983.

65. Fogler, W. E. and Fidler, I. J., Nonselective destruction of murine neoplastic cells by syngeneic tumoricidal macrophages, *Cancer Res.*, 45, 14, 1985.

66. Mantovani, A., Peri, G., Polentarutti, N., Bolis, G., Mangioni, C., and Spreafico, F., Effects on "in vitro" tumor growth of macrophages isolated from human ascitic ovarian tumors, *Int. J. Cancer*, 23, 157, 1979.

67. Haskill, S., Koren, H., Becker, S., Fowler, W., and Walton, L., Mononuclear cell infiltration in ovarian cancer. III. Suppressor-cell and ADCC activity or macrophages from ascitic and solid ovarian tumours, *Br. J. Cancer*, 45, 747, 1982.

68. Adams, D. O., Hall, T., Steplewski, Z., and Koprowski, H., Tumors undergoing rejection induced by monoclonal antibodies of the IgG2a isotype contain increased numbers of macrophages activated for a distinctive form of antibody-dependent cytolysis, *Proc. Natl. Acad. Sci. U.S.A.*, 81, 3506, 1984.

69. Estes, J. E., Pledger, W. J., and Gillespie, G. Y., Macrophage-derived growth factor for fibroblasts and interleukin-1 are distinct entities, *J. Leukocyte Biol.,* 35, 115, 1984.

70. Mantovani, A., Polentarutti, N., Peri, G., Bar Shavit, Z., Vecchi, A., Bolis, G., and Mangioni, C., Cytotoxicity on tumor cells of peripheral blood monocytes and tumor-associated macrophages in patients with ascites ovarian tumors, *J. Natl. Cancer Inst.,* 64, 1307, 1980.

71. Buick, R. N., Fry, S. E., and Salmon, S. E., Effect of host-cell interactions of clonogenic carcinoma cells in human malignant effusions, *Br. J. Cancer,* 41, 695, 1980.

72. Welander, C. E., Natale, R. B., and Lewis, J. L., Jr., In vitro growth stimulation of human ovarian cancer cells by xenogeneic peritoneal macrophages, *J. Natl. Cancer Inst.,* 69, 1039, 1982.

73. Gabizon, A., Leibovich, S. J., and Goldman, R., Contrasting effects of activated and nonactivated macrophages and macrophages from tumor-bearing mice on tumor growth in vivo, *J. Natl. Cancer Inst.,* 65, 913, 1980.

74. Nelson, M., Nelson, D. S., and Hopper, K. E., Inflammation and tumor growth. I. Tumor growth in mice with depressed capacity to mount inflammatory responses: possible role of macrophages, *Am. J. Pathol.,* 104, 114, 1981.

75. Evans, R., Macrophage requirement for growth of a murine fibrosarcoma, *Br. J. Cancer,* 37, 1086, 1978.

76. Evans, R., Duffy, T., and Cullen, R. T., Tumor-associated macrophages stimulate the proliferation of murine tumor cells surviving treatment with the oncolytic cyclophosphamide analogue Asta Z-7557: in vivo implications, *Int. J. Cancer,* 34, 883, 1984.

77. Kadhim, S. A. and Rees, R. C., Enhancement of tumor growth in mice: evidence for the involvement of host macrophages, *Cell. Immunol.,* 87, 259, 1984.

78. De Baetselier, P., Kapon, A., Katzav, S., Tzehoval, E., Dekegel, D., Segal, S., and Feldman, M., Selecting, accelerating and suppressing interactions between macrophages and tumor cells, *Invasion Met.,* 5, 106, 1985.

79. Lorenzet, R., Peri, G., Locati, D., Allavena, P., Colucci, M., Semeraro, N., Mantovani, A., and Donati, M. B., Generation of procoagulant activity by mononuclear phagocytes: a possible mechanism contributing to blood clotting activation within malignant tissues, *Blood,* 62, 271, 1983.

80. Guarini, A., Acero, R., Alessio, G., Donati, M. B., Semeraro, N., and Mantovani, A., Procoagulant activity of macrophages associated with different murine neoplasms, *Int. J. Cancer,* 34, 581, 1984.

81. Rambaldi, A., Alessio, G., Casali, B., Gambacorti-Passerini, C., Donati, M. B., Mantovani, A., and Semeraro, N., Induction of monocyte-macrophage procoagulant activity by transformed cell lines, *J. Immunol.,* in press.

82. Dvorak, H. F., Senger, D. R., and Dvorak, A. M., Fibrin as a component of the tumor stroma: origins and biological significance, *Cancer Met. Rev.,* 2, 41, 1983.

83. Rickles, F. R. and Edwards, R. L., Activation of blood coagulation in cancer: trousseau's syndrome revisited, *Blood,* 62, 14, 1983.

84. Nathan, C. F., The release of hydrogen peroxide from mononuclear phagocytes and its role in extracellular cytolysis, in *Mononuclear Phagocytes, Functional Aspects,* Van Furth, R., Ed., Martinus Nijhoff, Hingham, Mass., 1980, 1165.

85. Weitzman, S. A. and Stossel, T. P., Mutation caused by human phagocytes, *Science,* 212, 546, 1981.

86. Weitberg, A. B., Weitzman, S. A., Destrempes, M., Latt, S. A., and Stossel, T. P., Stimulated human phagocytes produce cytogenetic changes in cultured mammalian cells, *N. Engl. J. Med.,* 308, 26, 1983.

87. Fulton, A. M., Loveless, S. E., and Heppner, G., Mutagenic activity of tumor-associated macrophages in Salmonella typhimurium strains TA98 and TA100, *Cancer Res.,* 44, 4308, 1984.

88. Henry, N., van Lamsweerde, A-L., and Vaes, G., Collagen degradation by metastatic cells and macrophages, *Cancer Res.,* 43, 5321, 1983.

89. Folkman, J., What is the role of endothelial cells in angiogenesis?, *Lab. Invest.,* 51, 601, 1984.

90. Rossi, V., Breviario, F., Ghezzi, P., Dejana, E., and Mantovani, A., Interleukin-1 induces prostacyclin synthesis in vascular cells, *Science,* 229, 174, 1985.

91. Polverini, P. J., Cotran, R. S., Gimbrone, M. A., Jr., and Unanue, E. R., Activated macrophages induced vascular proliferation, *Nature (London),* 269, 804, 1977.

92. Polverini, P. J. and Leibovich, S. J., Induction of neovascularization in vivo and endothelial proliferation in vitro by tumor-associated macrophages, *Lab. Invest.,* 51, 635, 1984.

93. Peri, G., Polentarutti, N., Sessa, C., Mangioni, C., and Mantovani, A., Tumoricidal activity of macrophages isolated from human ascitic and solid ovarian carcinomas: augmentation by interferon lymphokines and endotoxin, *Int. J. Cancer,* 28, 143, 1981.

94. Haskill, S., Koren, H., Becker, S., Fowler, W., and Walton, L., Mononuclear-cell infiltration in ovarian cancer. III. Suppressor-cell and ADCC activity of macrophages from ascitic and solid ovarian tumours, *Br. J. Cancer,* 45, 747, 1982.

95. Rhodes, J., Plowman, P., Bishop, M., and Lipscomb, D., Human macrophage function in cancer: systemic and local changes detected by an assay of Fc receptor expression, *J. Natl. Cancer Inst.*, 66, 423, 1981.

96. Steele, R. J., Eremin, O., and Brown, M., Blood monocytes and tumor-infiltrating macrophages in human breast cancer: differences in activation level as assessed by lysozyme content, *J. Natl. Cancer Inst.*, 71, 941, 1983.

97. Steele, R. J., Brown, M., and Eremin, O., Characterization of macrophages infiltrating human mammary carcinomas, *Br. J. Cancer*, 51, 135, 1985.

98. Hammerstrom, J., Structure and function of human effusion macrophages from patients with malignant and benign disease. I. Isolation, morphology, proliferation and phagocytosis, *Acta Pathol. Microbiol. Scand. Sect. C*, 88, 191, 1980.

99. Hammerstrom, J., Structure and function of human effusion macrophages from patients with malignant and benign disease. II. In vitro cytostatic and cytolitic effect on human tumour cell lines, *Acta Pathol. Microbiol. Scand. Sect. C*, 88, 201, 1980.

100. Vose, B. M., Cytotoxicity of adherent cells associated with some human tumours and lung tissues, *Cancer Immunol. Immunother.*, 5, 173, 1978.

101. Colotta, F., Peri, G., Villa, A., and Mantovani, A., Rapid killing of actinomycin D-treated tumor cells by human mononuclear cells. I. Effectors belong to the monocyte-macrophage lineage, *J. Immunol.*, 132, 936, 1984.

102. Sherlock, P. and Hartman, W. H., Adrenal steroids and the pattern of metastases in breast cancer, *J. Am. Med. Assoc.*, 181.

103. Iversen, H. J. and Hjort, G. H., The influence of glucocorticoid steroids on the frequency of spleen metastases in patients with breast cancer, *Acta Pathol. Microbiol. Scand.*, 44, 205, 1958.

104. Fidler, I. J., Inhibition of pulmonary metastasis by intravenous injection of specifically activated macrophages, *Cancer Res.*, 34, 1074, 1976.

105. Den Otter, W., Dullens, F. J., Van Loveren, H., and Pels, E., Antitumor effects of macrophages injected into animals: a review, in *The Macrophage and Cancer*, James, K., McBride, B., and Stuart, A., Eds., Econoprint, Edinburgh, 1977, 119.

106. Gorelik, E., Wiltrout, R. H., Brunda, M. J., Holden, H. T., and Herberman, R. B., Augmentation of metastasis formation by thioglycollate-elicited macrophages, *Int. J. Cancer*, 29, 575, 1982.

107. Gorelik, E., Wiltrout, R. H., Copeland, D., and Herberman, R. B., Modulation of formation of tumor metastases by peritoneal macrophages elicited by various agents, *Cancer Immunol. Immunother.*, 19, 35, 1985.

108. Meltzer, M. S., Tumor cytotoxicity by lymphokine-activated macrophages: development of macrophage tumoricidal activity requires a sequence of reactions, in *Lymphokines*, Vol. 3, Pick, E., Ed., Academic Press, New York, 1981, 319.

109. Vose, B. M., Vanky, F., Argov, S., and Klein, E., Natural cytotoxicity in man: activity of lymph node and tumor-infiltrating lymphocytes, *eur. J. Immunol.*, 7, 753, 1977.

110. Mantovani, A., Allavena, P., Sessa, C., Bolis, G., and Mangioni, C., Natural killer activity of lymphoid cells isolated from human ascitic ovarian tumors, *Int. J. Cancer*, 25, 573, 1980.

111. Uchida, A. and Micksche, M., Natural killer cells in carcinomatus pleural effusions, *Cancer Immunol. Immunother.*, 11, 131, 1981.

112. Haskill, S., Koren, H., Becker, S., Fowler, W., and Walton, L., Mononuclear-cell infiltration in ovarian cancer. II. Immune function of tumor and ascites-derived inflammatory cells, *Br. J. Cancer*, 45, 737, 1982.

113. Berek, J. S., Bast, R. C., Jr., Lichtenstein, A., Hacker, N. F., Spina, C. A., Lagasse, L. D., Knapp, R. C., and Zighelboim, J., Lymphocyte cytotoxicity in the peritoneal activity and blood of patients with ovarian cancer, *Obstet. Gynecol.*, 64, 708, 1984.

114. Uchida, A. and Micksche, M., Suppressor cells for natural killer activity in carcinomatous pleural effusions of cancer patients, *Cancer Immunol. Immunother.*, 11, 255, 1981.

115. Uchida, A., Colot, M., and Micksche, M., Suppression of natural killer cell activity by adherent effusion cells of cancer patients. Suppression of motility, binding capacity and lethal hit of NK cells, *Br. J. Cancer*, 49, 17, 1984.

116. Introna, M., Allavena, P., Biondi, A., Colombo, N., Villa, A., and Mantovani, A., Defective natural killer activity within human ovarian tumors: low numbers of morphologically defined effectors are present in situ, *J. Natl. Cancer Inst.*, 70, 21, 1983.

117. Bhan, A. K. and DesMarais, C. L., Immunohistologic characterization of major histocompatibility antigens and inflammatory cellular infiltrate in human breast cancer, *J. Natl. Cancer Inst.*, 71, 507, 1983.

118. Eremin, O., Coombs, R. R. A., and Ashby, J., Lymphocytes infiltrating human breast cancers lack k-cell activity and show low levels of NK-cell activity, *Br. J. Cancer*, 44, 166, 1981.

119. Kabawat, S. E., Bast, R. C., Jr., Welch, W. R., Knapp, R. C., and Bhan, A. K., Expression of major histocompatibility antigens and nature of inflammatory cellular infiltrate in ovarian neoplasms, *Int. J. Cancer,* 32, 547, 1983.

120. Moy, P. M., Holmes, E. C., and Golub, S. H., Depression of natural killer cytotoxic activity in lymphocytes infiltrating human pulmonary tumors, *Cancer Res.,* 45, 57, 1985.

121. Hayry, P., Intragraft events in allograft destruction, *Transplantation,* 38, 1, 1984.

122. Bottazzi, B., Introna, M., Allavena, P., Villa, A., and Mantovani, A., In vitro migration of human large granular lymphocytes, *J. Immunol.,* 134, 2316, 1985.

123. Klein, E., Lymphocyte-mediated lysis of tumour cells in vitro. Antigen-restricted clonal and unrestricted polyclonal effects, *Springer Semin. Immunopathol.,* 5, 147, 1982.

124. Vose, B. M., Vanky, F., and Klein, E., Human tumour-lymphocyte interaction in vitro. V. Comparison of the reactivity of tumour-infiltrating, blood and lymph-node lymphocytes with autologous tumour cells, *Int. J. Cancer,* 20, 895, 1977.

125. Vose, B. M., Vanky, F., and Klein, E., Lymphocyte cytotoxicity against autologous tumour biopsy cells in humans, *Int. J. Cancer,* 20, 512, 1977.

126. Vose, B. M., Vanky, F., Fopp, M., and Klein, E., Restricted autologous lymphocytotoxicity in lung neoplasia, *Br. J. Cancer.,* 38, 375, 1978.

127. Allavena, P., IOntrona, M., Sessa, C., Mangioni, C., and Mantovani, A., Interferon effect on cytotoxicity of peripheral blood and tumor-associated lymphocytes against human ovarian carcinoma cells, *J. Natl. Cancer Inst.,* 68, 555, 1982.

128. Vanky, F., Willems, J., Kreicbergs, A., Aparisi, T., Andreen, M., Brostrom, L-A., Nilsonne, U., Klein, E., and Klein, G., Correlation between lymphocyte-mediated auto-tumor reactivities and clinical course. I. Evaluation of 46 patients with sarcoma, *Cancer Immunol. Immunother.,* 16, 11, 1983.

129. Vanky, F., Peterffy, A., Book, K., Willems, J., Klein, E., and Klein, G., Correlation between lymphocyte-mediated auto-tumor reactivities and the clinical course. II. Evaluation of 69 patients with lung carcinoma, *Cancer Immunol. Immunother.,* 16, 17, 1983.

130. Vose, B. M., Gallagher, P., Moore, M., and Schofield, P. F., Specific and non-specific lymphocyte cytotoxicity in colon carcinoma, *Br. J. Cancer,* 44, 846, 1981.

131. Vose, B. M., Quantitation of proliferative and cytotoxic precursor cells directed against human tumours: limiting dilution analysis in peripheral blood and at the tumour site, *Int. J. Cancer,* 30, 135, 1982.

132. Vose, B. M. and Moore, M., Suppressor cell activity of lymphocytes infiltrating human lung and breast tumours, *Int. J. Cancer,* 24, 579, 1979.

133. Buessow, S. C., Paul, R. D., Miller, A. M., and Lopez, D. M., Lymphoreticular cells isolated by centrifugal elutriation from a mammary adenocarcinoma. I. Characterization of an in situ lymphocyte suppressor population by surface markers and functional reactivity, *Int. J. Cancer,* 33, 79, 1984.

134. Mantovani, A., Bottazzi, B., Allavena, P., and Balotta, C., Unpublished data.

135. Mussonie, L. et al., Unpublished data.

INDEX

V

Variants, see also specific types

H2, 29
high-metastatic, 27, 45
Viruses, see also specific types
   lactic dehydrogenase elevating (LDV), 87